095876
D1628157

CHANGING CON
OF MOTHERHOOD
The Practice of Surrogacy in Britain

:TREET,
﹁ᴅ

ST. HELENS COMMUNITY LIBRARIES

3 8055 00473 9587

CHANGING CONCEPTIONS OF MOTHERHOOD
The Practice of Surrogacy in Britain

306-87

Published by the British Medical Association
Tavistock Square, London WC1H 9JP
January 1996

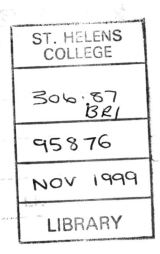

ST. HELENS
COLLEGE

306.87
BRI

95876

NOV 1999

LIBRARY

© British Medical Association 1996

All rights reserved. No part of this publication may be reproduced,
stored in a retrieval system, or transmitted, in any form or by any
means, electronic, mechanical, photocopying, recording and/or
otherwise, without prior permission of the publishers.

First printed in 1996

British Library Cataloguing Publication Data
A catalogue record for this book is available from the British Library

ISBN 0 7279 1006 X

Typeset in Great Britain by Apek Typesetters Ltd., Nailsea, Bristol.
Printed and bound by Latimer Trend and Co. Ltd., Plymouth, Devon.

Contents

Acknowledgements

We wish to thank the following for their assistance with the preparation of this report: Mr Eric Blyth, Dr Peter Brinsden, COTS (Childlessness Overcome Through Surrogacy), the Ethics Committee of the Royal College of Obstetricians and Gynaecologists and Dr John Parsons. Thanks are also due to other individuals and organisations who kindly offered advice and information for the report.

Membership of the Steering Group

Mr Derek Morgan, Chairman	Cardiff Law School; Member BMA Medical Ethics Committee
Ms Alison Britton	Lawyer, Glasgow University Institute of Law & Ethics in Medicine
Ms Jenny Clifford	Infertility Counsellor; British Infertility Counselling Association
Dr Rachel Cook	Chartered Psychologist, King's College, London
Dr Roger Crisp	Fellow in Philosophy, St Anne's College, Oxford
Ms Veronica English	Senior Research Officer, BMA Medical Ethics Department
Dr Ruth Gilbert	Paediatrician; Member BMA Medical Ethics Committee
Mr Anthony Nysenbaum	Consultant Obstetrician & Gynaecologist; Royal College of Obstetricians & Gynaecologists
Ms Dora Opoku	Head of Midwifery Education, Royal College of Midwives
Dr Frances Price	Sociologist, University of Cambridge Centre for Family Research
Dr Anne Rodway	General Practitioner; Member BMA Medical Ethics Committee
Ms Ann Sommerville	Advisor to the BMA on Medical Ethics

Observer

Ms Jennifer Woodside	Human Fertilisation & Embryology Authority

Contributing Authors
Ms Alison Britton
Dr Rachel Cook
Dr Roger Crisp
Ms Veronica English
Ms Ann Sommerville

Editor:	Mr Derek Morgan
Head of Division:	Dr Fleur Fisher
Project Manager:	Miss Rosemary Weston

Preface

Over the last twenty years a revolution has taken place in the field of human reproduction. The development of techniques like in vitro fertilisation and our increased understanding of the earliest stages of human development have opened up new opportunities for those unable to have children in the usual way. Surrogacy is one such opportunity. The number of people using surrogacy is small in comparison with those using other forms of assisted reproduction but, in many ways, it raises more profound questions and challenges some of our most deeply held beliefs. The separation of maternity from social motherhood raises complex issues but some studies appear to show increasing support for this method of overcoming childlessness. Part of this apparent growing acceptance is likely to be linked to the amount of publicity given to surrogacy over the last few years with increasing numbers of human interest stories relating to surrogacy arrangements. However, these stories almost invariably portray only the positive side of surrogacy. Less frequently are the tragic cases exposed for public viewing. In those which are reported, such as the rare cases where the surrogate decides to keep the child, the pain and distress caused is undeniable.

The BMA's views on surrogacy have changed over time. From advice to doctors to have no involvement with surrogacy, came a growing recognition that surrogacy is as much a social issue as a medical one. This recognition led to the BMA's acceptance of surrogacy as a treatment of last resort. The Association's last report on surrogacy was published in 1990, in response to a mandate from the BMA's Annual Representative Meeting. There are a number of reasons why it was considered that the time is now ripe for this guidance to be reassessed and for further guidance to be issued. One reason is the apparent growing public acceptance of surrogacy and changing attitudes in society generally about this practice. This has led to a reduction in the amount of secrecy surrounding the practice and to a corresponding increase in the number of people requesting advice and support from the medical profession about surrogacy arrangements. This guidance therefore seeks to reflect changing attitudes about surrogacy as well as changes in the law and in practice.

But this is not the only reason for addressing the issue now. Despite the problems predicted by some people, evidence appears to suggest that surrogacy in Britain has been less fraught with disputes than in other countries. Patients are now, more than ever, travelling to other parts of the world for treatment which is either unavailable or is legally prohibited in their own country and infertility treatment provides a very clear example of this. As the ease of travel around the world increases, and restrictive legislation is introduced in more countries, this form of "medical tourism" is likely to increase. This means that we must look not only to Britain but also to the practices in other countries so that the type of disputes and exploitation we see in some other parts of the world can be avoided. During 1995, there were two press reports of the use of women from Eastern Europe as surrogate mothers for wealthy western couples. Plans were reported, of a scheme to take women from such countries as Poland, Romania and Hungary to Germany, Holland, Belgium, America and Canada. According to one report the women were to be paid for their services, having been smuggled to the west under the guise of working as au pairs, and in the other, the intention was to take women to America to give birth which, in certain states, would entitle them to American citizenship. Counselling, support, legal advice and medical follow-up are not built into these kinds of schemes. It is the fear of this type of exploitation of economically or socially vulnerable women which has led to a complete ban on surrogacy in some countries such as France. The Federal Government of Canada has announced a voluntary moratorium on a number of reproductive technologies including commercial surrogacy. They are now looking at the regulation of such technologies in order to ensure that such exploitation can be avoided. It is hoped that this report, and the guidelines contained within it, together with the existing regulatory framework, will increase awareness and minimise the possibility of abuse in Britain.

Introduction

Background

Despite the absence of official figures, evidence from a variety of sources clearly suggests that surrogacy arrangements are increasing in Britain. The practice of surrogacy, where one woman agrees to bear a child for another and surrender it at birth, provides an opportunity for women for whom pregnancy is medically impossible or highly undesirable to circumvent their childlessness and become a mother to a child. Fears of exploitation, concern about unknown psychological and other health risks and anxiety about the way children might come to be seen as commodities, mean that surrogacy is widely regarded by health professionals and the public as a reproductive option of last resort. Nevertheless, public awareness and acceptance of surrogacy appears to be growing for those cases where all other measures have failed[1]. Although reports of public opinion should be received with due caution, media coverage of infertility generally, and surrogacy specifically, has increased the general level of understanding of the issues involved. Although some regret this, notions about what constitutes normality for "the family" are also changing, as arrangements previously regarded as unconventional become more common. This report endeavours to ensure that the apparently increasing acceptance of surrogacy is accompanied by an awareness of both the benefits and risks.

In Parliament opinion on surrogacy appears double-edged. The Surrogacy Arrangements Act 1985 reacted to public concern at the time by outlawing commercial surrogacy agencies. It did not prohibit voluntary agencies facilitating surrogacy arrangements nor did it prohibit payments to surrogate mothers. Surrogacy arrangements were declared legally unenforceable by the Human Fertilisation and Embryology Act 1990. The same Act, however, simplified the procedure for transferring legal parentage of a surrogate born child, ensuring that where the people who intend to raise the child have also donated their gametes for its creation, they can be recognised as parents in law. This may be taken to imply a certain acceptance of surrogacy.

1

The Human Fertilisation and Embryology Act also established the Human Fertilisation & Embryology Authority (HFEA) as the regulatory body for licensing certain types of fertility treatment and research. Although surrogacy is not a regulated activity, where health professionals provide fertility treatment which involves either the creation of embryos outside the body or the donation of eggs or sperm (as with insemination for a surrogacy arrangement), they are bound by HFEA guidelines. They are also legally obliged to take account of the welfare of any child likely to be born, or affected, by the treatment.

BMA Policy

The BMA acknowledges surrogacy as a reproductive option of last resort, in which the interests of the potential child must be paramount. It maintains the widely accepted view that surrogacy should only be considered when it is impossible or highly undesirable for medical reasons for the intended mother to carry a child herself. The BMA opposes the use of surrogacy arrangements for social reasons or for convenience and notes that there is no evidence of this occurring in Britain. A prime consideration for health professionals, in addition to the welfare of the potential child, is that the risks to the surrogate mother must be minimised and that her wishes about the conduct of the pregnancy take precedence over those of the other adults involved.

In its 1990 report, *Surrogacy: Ethical Considerations*, the BMA recommended that surrogacy arrangements should be made and conducted anonymously (see section 3:7). This advice was based largely on concerns about the psychological health of the surrogate mother and the child. However, information collected, about current practice, during the preparation of this report does not appear to support these concerns. Furthermore, experience suggests that contact between the surrogate mother and the intended parents is preferred by many participants and can have a positive effect for all concerned. It is now clear that anonymity is not necessarily a desirable or realistic option in every case. The BMA now advises that decisions on this matter should be made on an individual and well informed basis by the people involved.

Over a number of years, the BMA has received reports indicating that some people enter into surrogacy arrangements with insufficient information or advice about the legal, medical and emotional aspects of their decision. They potentially expose themselves and others to avoidable distress. Before initiating a surrogacy arrangement, the BMA considers it vital that those considering surrogacy or advising others about it should have access to relevant and accurate information.

Where assisted conception techniques are used, health professionals providing treatment services are required to supply information, but indicators suggest that in a high proportion of surrogacy cases medical advice is not sought. For those who do not consult health professionals, the main source of information and advice appears to be voluntary surrogacy agencies. At present these agencies are unregulated and unmonitored. While it is clear that many of the individuals involved in these voluntary bodies are dedicated and conscientious, there is no formal mechanism for ensuring that the information they provide concerning what are increasingly complex issues of law and medicine is accurate or comprehensive. Nor is there any safety net if such agencies find themselves overstretched; because they are forbidden by law from charging for their services, their access to expert legal and other support is limited. While the BMA does not propose a formal system of licensing voluntary agencies, it believes that some form of monitoring would be highly desirable, both from the public interest perspective and to ensure the credibility of the voluntary agencies.

The BMA is also concerned about the lack of opportunity for medical and psychological support for individuals involved in surrogacy arrangements. The type and degree of support which could usefully be accessed can only be a matter of speculation in the absence of monitoring of the type of health or other problems which arise. Information concerning the welfare of the children or the long-term effects on surrogate mothers, their other children and the intended parents is only generally available from voluntary agencies and clinics which support surrogacy, or by extrapolation from cognate studies. Even then, the information is largely unsystematic and anecdotal. While the lack of such data might be thought to indicate that arrangements do not generate particular problems, there is no means of measuring whether cases which tragically go wrong are exceptional or symptomatic of wider difficulties. A danger exists that policies and debate rely on myth and supposition rather than fact. This report gathers together the limited information available and augments the BMA's guidance for health professionals.

This Report

This report updates the BMA's 1990 report. Since then there have been changes in law and practice as well as in apparent public tolerance. The background to the current surrogacy debate is summarised in chapter 1. The law, ethics and current practice are discussed in chapters 2 and 3. Medical aspects which should be known by the participants in a surrogacy arrangement are raised in chapter 4. Analysis of the psychological implications which surrogacy may hold for the various parties is extremely complex, not least due to the difficulties of examining a practice which is largely unmonitored. Chapter 5 brings together such data and opinions as are available. Counselling is rightly seen as a vital component of any kind of fertility treatment and the importance of access to counselling, including for individuals who choose not to use fertility clinics or other health facilities for surrogacy, is discussed in chapter 6. Chapter 7 provides a summary of the issues in the form of practical guidance for health professionals. Some repetition in the text is unavoidable and is indeed desirable since it is expected that many health professionals will dip into the chapters as they are relevant to particular enquiries rather than read the book from cover to cover.

Surrogacy is one way, and for some people the only practical way, of addressing the consequences of involuntary childlessness. This report provides such information as is available about the demand for surrogacy and the various forms it takes. The practice of surrogacy raises questions of social interest far beyond the scope of health professionals to resolve. Nevertheless, doctors, nurses, midwives and health visitors have particular moral responsibilities both to the adults they care for and the children born as a result of medical treatment. The role of professional bodies like the BMA must be to provide guidance for their own members and their colleagues as a contribution towards promoting enlightened public debate and well informed decisions by individuals.

1 The Practice of Surrogacy

1:1 Terms Used in the Report

Surrogate: The term surrogate mother or surrogate is used throughout this report to refer to the woman who carries and delivers the baby. Whilst this is in line with common usage it is not without difficulty. Some commentators argue that it is the woman who rears the child rather than the one who gives birth to it, who is the *surrogate* mother and that the woman who gives birth is *the* mother not the surrogate. This argument is given further weight by the fact that the woman who bears the child is its initial legal mother (see section 2:4). Other commentators propose that the surrogate is a substitute for maternity, not motherhood, and that popular usage properly reflects this[2]. (The different forms of surrogacy are defined in section 1:3.)

Intended parents: This term refers to those who, under a surrogacy arrangement, will be the social parents of the child, or who, following adoption or a "parental order" (see section 2:5), will be the social and legal parents of the child. Traditionally, the term "commissioning couple" had been used but this is gradually being replaced in the literature by intending or intended parents more accurately to reflect the nature of the agreement made and to remove elements of commercial taint attaching to the earlier description. The term intended parents, therefore, has been used throughout this report to refer to those who previously have been known as the commissioning couple.

Parents: In this context, the plural term "parents" is used but this is not intended to prejudge or limit who might be eligible or fit for raising children. Indeed as the Warnock Committee[3] made clear, judgments about such matters go far beyond purely medical considerations. The BMA's recorded view has long been that careful consideration must be given to the circumstances of each family, the needs of the individuals involved, and most importantly the welfare of any child who might be born as a result of fertility treatment. This view is reinforced by legal provisions which do not exclude from fertility services less traditional family arrangements but oblige treatment providers to consider the child's welfare and in particular its need for a father. Nevertheless, other constraints exist which, in practice, tend to restrict those contemplating surrogacy to heterosexual couples. In order to apply for a parental order, for example, applicants must be married to one another. The alternative procedure for establishing legal parenthood, by adoption, favours those in stable heterosexual relationships. Without venturing into wider social and moral arguments, practical requirements appear to make it preferable for a surrogacy arrangement to involve two parents who together intend to raise the child. It is important to stress, however, that people in diverse types of family arrangement are not excluded from seeking medical advice, services or counselling.

1:2 Childlessness

The incidence of childlessness is notoriously difficult to calculate. Many people make a positive choice to remain childless whereas others may wish to have children but experience difficulty conceiving. Studies have suggested that between 1 in 6 and 1 in 8 couples in the UK have fertility problems. It has been argued that the proportion has changed little over the years but that the incidence is now becoming more visible as more people seek medical assistance to overcome the consequences of their infertility. Recent literature, however, has suggested that the amount of infertility, particularly male infertility, has actually increased.

Many couples are childless because the egg and sperm do not combine to make an embryo. There are multiple reasons for this, the most common being poor quality sperm or blocked fallopian tubes. In some cases, however, there is no obvious cause. Techniques such as in vitro fertilisation (IVF) can be used to try to overcome these types of infertility by collecting the egg and sperm and placing them together under laboratory conditions to fertilise. The resulting embryos are then replaced in the uterus. Other methods of assisted reproduction can also be used.

For some people, the problem is not one of contributing to the creation of an embryo, but of the woman carrying the resulting fetus to term. A variety of causes account for this, including failure of the embryo to implant, repeated miscarriage, hysterectomy or a pelvic disorder. Some women experience problems such as dangerously high blood pressure, a heart condition or liver disease, so that pregnancy entails a serious health risk for them.

Coming to terms with childlessness may be an acceptable option for some people, or a regretted inevitability. Adoption or fostering may offer an acceptable alternative, but the number of people wishing to pursue this option vastly outnumber the babies and children available in Britain. Surrogacy may be seen as a possible solution. Conjecture sometimes focuses on hypothetical examples of women who want children, are perfectly capable of pregnancy and childbirth but who wish to avoid the physical, social, psychological or financial drawbacks of bearing a child themselves. If this were shown to be a realistic concern, the BMA would oppose women being exposed to the health risks associated with IVF and pregnancy to save others the inconvenience. Doubt might also be cast on the future well-being of any child born into such a situation. It is unlikely, however, given all the uncertainties which accompany surrogacy, that informed parties on either side enter into it for such superficial reasons. The experience of health professionals and others involved with surrogacy indicate that such "social" requests are highly unusual.

1:3 Surrogacy

Distinction can be made between "partial" surrogacy (also known as traditional or straight surrogacy) and "full" surrogacy (also known as host or IVF surrogacy). In partial surrogacy the surrogate mother provides an egg which is fertilised with sperm from the intended father, or a donor, by insemination, in vitro fertilisation or another form of assisted reproduction. On rare occasions, pregnancy results from sexual intercourse with the intended father. Some people see partial surrogacy as an alternative to egg donation in cases where the intended mother cannot produce eggs but would be capable of carrying a child to term. However, the BMA considers it unacceptable to subject another woman to the risks of pregnancy when other treatment options, such as egg donation, are medically possible. Therefore surrogacy should only be considered in cases where there are no other treatment alternatives.

In full surrogacy the woman who carries the fetus makes no genetic contribution to an embryo which she receives to gestate. The eggs and sperm used to create the embryo are usually those of the intended parents, although in some cases donated gametes may be used. For example if the intended mother, in addition to being unable to carry the fetus, is also unable to produce eggs, an alternative to partial surrogacy is to use donated eggs for IVF and subsequent replacement of the embryo into the surrogate mother.

1:4 Incidence of Surrogacy

Although various ways of estimating the extent of surrogacy in Britain have been tried, it is currently impossible to know the real incidence of surrogacy arrangements. Some arrangements are made secretly between family members or friends. Section 30 of the Human Fertilisation and Embryology Act, which came into effect on 1 November 1994, allows intended parents to apply to a competent court to transfer the parentage of the child in surrogacy cases. Measuring the number of such applications might provide a means of assessing the extent of some types of surrogacy at a particular time. These parental orders are applicable only under some carefully defined conditions (the intended parents must be married to each other at the time of the application, for example, and one of them must have donated gametes to the child, see section 2:5) so even an analysis of all parental orders at a given time does not necessarily indicate the full extent of surrogacy although it provides a useful indicator.

In 1995, a study of applications lodged for parental orders in the immediate six month period from 1 November 1994 - 30 April 1995 was commissioned for this report. It tried to gauge the incidence of surrogacy, based on the assumption that parents who had had a surrogate born child at any time in the past might use this "retrospective window" (see section 2:5) to formalise the relationship, as contemplated by section 30. An analysis of orders successfully pursued showed, however, that fewer than 50 parties took this opportunity. Assuming that this does not represent the true incidence of surrogacy arrangements which may have stretched back for many years, a number of reasons might account for this.

Firstly some solicitors experienced in working with parties involved

8

in surrogacy cases reported that the different responses of court appointed guardians ad litem, (under the provisions of the Adoption Act 1976 (as amended) section 65 and the Adoption (Scotland) Act 1978 (as amended) section 58) to report on the suitability of the intended parents, and the delays experienced by some applicants, had persuaded others that the alternative route of the adoption procedure was a more valuable way to proceed. The adoption route was, they reported, likely to take no longer than that for parental orders, although there was clearly a wide divergence of experience, with some witnesses informing us that their section 30 application was processed in about a month while others complained of the bureaucratic and seemingly laborious manner adopted by some guardians ad litem. Of course, there may be a variety of reasons which would explain or account for these differences, and delays cannot always be assumed to be a fault to be attributed to the system or those who were charged with the onerous duty of seeking to ensure the welfare of the surrogate born child who was the subject of the application.

Secondly, it appears that some people were dissuaded from using the parental orders procedure because their legal advisers had pointed to what they believed to be the more secure effect of the successful pursuit of adoption, extinguishing as it does all previous parental rights and responsibility. Obviously, this would have had strong appeal for some couples in preference to a section 30 procedure, which, they were advised, did not appear to extinguish all parental responsibilities vesting in the surrogate mother.

It is clear, however, that the Parental Orders (Human Fertilisation and Embryology) Regulations 1994 (S.I. 1994/2767) and the Parental Orders (Human Fertilisation and Embryology) (Scotland) Regulations 1994 (S.I. 1994/2804) (made under the provisions of the Human Fertilisation and Embryology Act 1990, sections 30(9), 45(1) and (3)), are intended to achieve the same effect as an adoption order. The relevant provisions of those regulations are Paragraph 1(1), (2) and Paragraph 2, column 1, Schedule 1, sub-para. 1(b), which adopts (under section 30(9) of the 1990 Act) amended provisions of the Adoption Act 1976, section 12 (1)-(3), and in Scotland the equivalent provisions of the Adoption (Scotland) Act 1978. As amended, the relevant part of that section reads:

"(1) A parental order is an order giving parental responsibility for a child to the husband and wife, made on their application by an authorised court.

. . .

(3) The making of a parental order operates to extinguish:
(a) the parental responsibility which any person has for the child immediately before the making of the order;
(aa) any order under the Children Act 1989;
(b) any duty arising by virtue of an agreement or the order of a court to make payments, so far as the payments are in respect of the child's maintenance or upbringing for any period after the making of the order."

Insofar as some potential applicants may have been deterred from pursuing the section 30 route in the mistaken belief that the surrogate mother might have retained some rights in respect of the child, this misunderstanding is unfortunate.

Thirdly, in some families with a surrogate born child, one of the spouses may have died since the child's birth and delivery up to them, indeed in the course of this study evidence was provided of two such cases. The benefits of section 30 are afforded to "the parties to a marriage"; the death of either partner ends the marriage, and the sole surviving spouse is not, under the usual interpretation, entitled to make a parental order application. The same would be the case if the intended parents had since the birth of the child divorced. In the course of this study, information was provided of one case in which a parental order had been made in favour of an individual applicant whose spouse had died since the birth of the child (in circumstances unrelated to the surrogacy). It has been suggested that the legal effect of such an order may be worthless and it might be possible for the surrogate mother to seek rectification of the Parental Orders Register and seek to recover the child. If this is the case, the child could, until majority, seek support from the surrogate and, if she is married, her husband. If the parental order, as granted by the court is, in fact, worthless, the surviving spouse would need to seek an adoption order to be regarded, in law, as the parent of the child.

Fourthly, some couples who in the past have had a child born as a consequence of a surrogacy arrangement may have already successfully applied for adoption, or may have never revealed the fact of the surrogacy and registered the child at birth as though it was their child, or may have been unaware of the provisions of the 1990 Act and how it could have applied to their benefit. During the preparation of this report, the Steering Group were informed on a number of occasions of the anxiety shared by witnesses that, despite the best efforts of the Department of Health, and the Welsh and Scottish Offices, people who really needed to know of the existence of section 30 had been missed. Finally, some courts questioned about their experience with parental orders applications did not respond, and it is impossible to know whether any of these were courts in which an order had been sought or granted.

Thus, while the study was able to indicate some level of surrogacy activity, and some which had been previously unknown or unreported, it is clear that only a partial picture emerged. Yet it lends support to the view expressed in evidence of voluntary surrogacy agencies that the use and incidence of surrogacy in the UK is growing.

1:5 Surrogacy Agencies and the Provision of Information

Although commercial surrogacy agencies are illegal there is little restriction on voluntary agencies. They can give information, advice and support to those interested in surrogacy and put potential surrogate mothers and intended parents in touch with each other. As partial surrogacy does not require medical intervention this contact may, for some, be the only opportunity to obtain practical information, or advice about the services they need. Although they provide a public service unavailable elsewhere and arguably may provide the only practical means of providing long-term psychological support or evidence of the impact of surrogacy, these agencies work informally and are reliant upon the commitment and good will of a small number of members. They are unmonitored, unregulated and are themselves unsupported in any way by the state, since they are ineligible for charitable status and unable to charge for their services. There is no formal mechanism for ensuring that the information and advice they provide is accurate and comprehensive and no obvious way of ensuring that potential complaints are properly investigated, apart from costly and time consuming individual resort to the courts.

This is a matter of concern to the BMA. The Association believes it is essential that those involved in a surrogacy arrangement should have access to verifiable accurate information in order to make properly informed decisions. The Association advocates the introduction of some form of monitoring of the agencies and has urged the Department of Health to take up this issue.

2 Surrogacy and the Law

The legal approach to surrogacy in the United Kingdom has been piecemeal. Commercial surrogacy arrangements were prohibited by the Surrogacy Arrangements Act 1985, seen by one commentator as "a largely irrelevant panicked measure"[4]. This Act required neither monitoring nor minimum standards of conduct and expertise for the operation of non-commercial agencies. If the intended parents seek to adopt the child, this is governed by the Adoption Act 1976; a joint adoption order can only be made by and in favour of a married couple so that cohabiting intended parents could not both be made legal parents[5]. Additional provisions relevant to surrogacy were introduced in the Human Fertilisation and Embryology Act 1990.

A set of minimum statutory requirements for surrogacy advocated by a respected American commentator contain some basic provisions designed to secure and protect the interests of the child. None of these feature in our domestic law. The first is that obligatory medical screening of the participants in surrogacy arrangements should be introduced to minimise the risk of avoidable disease or disability. Secondly, if surrogacy was regarded as a form of prenatal adoption, so that the parties to the arrangement would be bound by normal parental obligations of care and support, this would reduce the likelihood of abandonment of the child, for example if born with a disability[6].

2:1 Surrogacy Arrangements Act 1985

The Surrogacy Arrangements Act 1985 (as amended), which is given in full as an appendix to this report, prohibits agencies or individuals (other than the potential surrogate mother or intended parents) from acting on a commercial basis to initiate, negotiate or compile information towards the making of a surrogacy arrangement. The Act prohibits any advertising (including by the potential surrogate mother or intended parents) which indicates that a person is willing to be a surrogate mother, that someone is looking for a surrogate mother or that a person or organisation will help to initiate a surrogacy arrangement. The Act does not, however, prohibit non-commercial agencies, or the activities of someone who

NEWTON LE WILLOWS
COMMUNITY LIBRARY
TEL: NLW 223729

might arrange a surrogacy non-commercially, nor does it prohibit payment to a surrogate mother.

2:2 Human Fertilisation and Embryology Act 1990

The Human Fertilisation & Embryology Authority (HFEA) was charged to regulate certain types of infertility treatment and research. It is a statutory requirement for a centre undertaking any of these activities to have a licence from the Authority which specifies the activities covered by the licence, the premises in which the activities may be performed and the name of a "person responsible" under whose supervision the work must be carried out[7]. Licensed activities include the creation or use of an embryo outside the body and the use of donated eggs, sperm or embryos. Medical treatments such as insemination, when used as part of a surrogacy arrangement, will involve the donation of sperm, eggs or embryos and thus must be carried out in a licensed centre. Under the Act's requirements, details of every treatment carried out must be lodged with the HFEA. Thus, although the Authority does not directly regulate surrogacy, licensed treatment services provided to establish a surrogate pregnancy will be carried out under its auspices.

2:3 Enforceability of Surrogacy Arrangements

Those participating in a surrogacy arrangement must reach agreement between themselves as to how the arrangement will proceed. Nevertheless, regardless of whether the agreement is detailed in writing or whether expenses have been paid, the Human Fertilisation and Embryology Act section 36 renders surrogacy contracts unenforceable[8]. This means that if the surrogate mother wishes to keep the child she is entitled to do so. Equally if the intended parents decide they do not want the child, the surrogate mother, as the legal mother of the child (see section 2:4), is responsible in law for its welfare. In practice, a child rejected by its birth mother and the intended parents is likely to be placed for fostering or adoption.

2:4 Legal Definitions of Mother and Father

Assisted reproduction techniques have required close definition of "mother", "father" and "parent". The 1990 Act provides a framework for these new status provisions. The basic principle of maternity is that the birth mother is the mother of the child, regardless of its genetic makeup[9]. The rules in relation to paternity are more complex, but may be summarised as follows[10]:

The child's father will be:

- the surrogate's husband - if she is married;
- the surrogate's partner - if she is not married, unless the partner can show that he did not consent to the treatment;
- the intended father - if the surrogate does not have a partner and the treatment did not take place at a centre licensed by the HFEA (ie. self-insemination).

The child will have no legal father if the treatment took place in a licensed centre and the surrogate does not have a partner[11].

If either party reneges on the agreement (which they may do), the surrogate mother, and if she has one, her partner, are legally responsible for the child. If the intended father is the legal father of the child (as defined above) and the surrogate mother decides to keep the child, it is possible that he would be liable to pay maintenance for the child. Questions concerning the legal parentage of the child should be explicitly addressed by all participants before a surrogacy arrangement is initiated.

2:5 Parental Orders

Section 30 of the Human Fertilisation and Embryology Act was brought into effect on 1 November 1994. This section provides that if a woman gives a child she has conceived to a married couple under a surrogacy arrangement, a competent court may make a "parental order". The effect of the order is to make the intended parents the child's legal parents. All applications will be reviewed by a court-appointed guardian ad litem, and the emphasis in the review will be placed on the best interests of the child in order to offer maximum protection. All proceedings are conducted in private.

There are a number of criteria which must be met before a parental order can be made.

- *The child must be genetically related to one or both of the intended parents;*
  The gametes (sperm or eggs) used in the child's conception must be those of one or both of the couple who intend to apply for a parental order. The guardian ad litem appointed to consider each case has the power to request DNA testing but it is likely that this power will only be used where there is a dispute between the parties to the agreement.

- *The intended parents must be married to each other and both be aged 18 or over;*
  This excludes couples who choose not to marry. It also excludes those whose marriage has ended before the making of the application, for example, through the death of one spouse, or following divorce. The marriage must be in existence at the time of the making of the section 30 parental order, and not merely at the initiation of the application.

- *The legal mother and father must consent to the making of a parental order;*
  The application must be made with the agreement of both the legal mother and father of the child (including a person who is the father by virtue of section 28 of the 1990 Act). Agreement must be given unconditionally and with the full understanding of what is involved, unless such persons cannot be found or are incapable of giving their agreement. This agreement cannot validly be given until six weeks after the birth of the child. This allows the surrogate mother time to reflect on her decision. It also allows her to change her mind, even if the child is already living with the intended parents.

- *No money other than reasonable expenses shall have been paid in respect of the surrogacy arrangement unless the payment has been authorised by a court;*
  The court must be satisfied that no money or other benefit has changed hands either for (i) the making of the parental order; (ii) the agreement to relinquish the child to the intended parents; (iii) the giving of the child to the applicants or (iv) for the making of the original surrogacy arrangement. There are two exceptions to

this prohibition; the court may sanction payments which have been made, and payment to the surrogate mother of "reasonable expenses" is permitted. The Act does not define what is to be regarded as reasonable expenses for this purpose.

- *Domicile;*
  At the time of the application, the child's home must be with the intended parents and one or both of them must be domiciled in a part of the United Kingdom or in the Channel Islands or the Isle of Man.

From November 1994 until April 1995, the Act opened a window for couples whose child was born at any time in the past following a surrogacy arrangement. Any married couple caring for a child born under such an arrangement, provided they met the other criteria, could apply for a parental order. For births after 1 November 1994 the application must be made within six months of the child's birth.

2:6 Birth Registration

A child born to a surrogate mother must be registered as her child, and if applicable, that of her partner or person treated as the father under the legislation. Where a parental order has been granted by a court, the Registrar General will make an entry in a separate Parental Order Register registering the child and cross referencing to the entry in the existing Register of Births. There is no public Parental Order Register. It is not possible to "abolish" the original record of birth and at the age of 18, a person who was the subject of a parental order may be supplied with information enabling him or her to obtain a certified copy of the original record of their birth. This certificate will include the name of the surrogate mother. Prior to being given access to the information the person is to be advised of counselling services available.

2:7 HFEA Code of Practice

The Human Fertilisation & Embryology Authority issues licences to centres carrying out certain activities. One aspect of the Authority's supervisory role is the publication of a Code of Practice which provides guidance concerning proper conduct of licensed activities.

All centres providing licensed treatment services (see section 2:2), for the purpose of establishing a surrogate pregnancy, must be licensed by the HFEA and abide by the Code of Practice.

One of the provisions of the 1990 Act makes it a condition of all treatment licences that "a woman shall not be provided with treatment services unless account has been taken of the welfare of any child who may be born as a result of the treatment (including the need of that child for a father), and of any other child who may be affected by the birth"[12].

Thus all centres providing licensed treatment services as part of a surrogacy arrangement are legally obliged to take account of the welfare of the child. This requirement is complicated by the fact that either the surrogate mother and her partner, if she has one, or the intended parents could take on the role of social parents; the centre is therefore obliged to make enquiries of both parties. The HFEA's Code of Practice advises consideration of the following factors:

- the commitment of the woman, and her husband/partner to having and bringing up a child or children;
- their ages and medical histories and the medical histories of their families;
- the needs of any child or children who may be born as a result of treatment, including the implications of any possible multiple birth and the ability of the prospective parents (or parent) to meet those needs;
- any risk of harm to the child or children who may be born, including the risk of inherited disorders, problems during pregnancy and of neglect or abuse; and
- the effect of a new baby on any existing child of the family[13].

The HFEA also advises in its Code of Practice that all people seeking treatment are entitled to a fair and unprejudiced assessment of their situation and needs, which should be conducted with the skill and sensitivity appropriate to the delicacy of the case and the wishes and feelings of those involved[14].

In addition, the Code sets an upper age limit for egg donors of 35 years because of the increased risk of chromosomal abnormalities with increasing age. With full surrogacy, the intended mother is considered, in law, to be the egg donor and therefore should be within this age limit. The Code of Practice allows for this limit to be exceeded if there are "exceptional reasons" for doing so but the reasons must be explained in the treatment records and the clinic must be prepared to justify its decision[15].

2:8 Legal Liabilities

Attempts could be made to take legal action against one or more of the participants in a surrogacy arrangement falling short of seeking to enforce the arrangement. It may be possible for a child to seek damages for negligence against the surrogate mother or the intended parents if they failed to seek appropriate testing for infectious diseases and the child is born with such a disease. The surrogate mother could attempt to sue the intended father if, through the insemination procedure, she contracted an infection such as HIV. The intended parents might seek to take legal action against a surrogate mother whose behaviour during the pregnancy led to the death or injury of the baby she was carrying. Such actions are likely to be very rare.

3 Ethical and Practical Considerations

3:1 The Ethics of Decision-making

The complexities and unpredictabilities of life mean that every case of surrogacy is different. The present report can only inform health professionals about some aspects of surrogacy which should be considered in every case. This is not to imply that health professionals carry the sole burden and responsibility of choice, rather that a primary part of their role is to help individuals make informed choices.

When health professionals provide treatment services to initiate a pregnancy, however, they have special ethical responsibilities for the outcome. They cannot see themselves simply as technicians carrying out the autonomous decisions of their patients. It is sometimes argued that health professionals cannot owe duties to potential people who may never come into existence and therefore that ethical responsibilities for the child only crystallise at birth. A counter view is that by disregarding the implications of present actions for people yet unborn, individuals become self-seeking and society is diminished. The clear message in this report, as with others published by the BMA, is that health professionals are bound both legally and ethically to consider the welfare of any child who may be born through their intervention in the provision of infertility treatment services.

This is not to imply that the ethical responsibilities of health professionals will necessarily conflict with those of other parties. On the contrary, evidence the BMA has taken in the course of compiling this report very clearly indicates that almost invariably all the parties to a surrogacy arrangement are preoccupied with the well-being of the child they hope will be born. There should be mutual trust and openness between health professionals and those who consult them, as much as between the individual parties to the arrangement. People are often alert to the possibility that realisation of their own desires may not ultimately be achievable or may, for some reason, not be the best for the other people involved, including the potential child. To come to terms with disappointment and accepting childlessness are particularly difficult within the social expectations of our society and the people involved may require support.

It is important that all of the participants in any arrangement, including the health professionals, do not disguise the fact that a great deal of stress, anxiety, pain, effort and money may be expended to no avail. It is advisable that health professionals and individuals make decisions jointly as carefully as possible, in full awareness of the narrow limits of what can be assured and giving due weight to each of the relevant factors.

3:2 Differing Levels of Professional Involvement

In surrogacy arrangements, health professionals incur differing levels of ethical responsibility concomitant with their degree of involvement in the arrangement. There are three broad categories of involvement.

3:2.1 An established pregnancy
When women present for antenatal and other care for an established surrogate pregnancy, the duty of the health care team is to provide the appropriate level of advice and care. Generally this would be the same care as required in any other pregnancy. In some cases, more information or support may be needed and if problems arise in the pregnancy, the anxieties are more diffuse. It also may be more complicated to ensure confidentiality for each individual involved in a surrogacy arrangement when several people all have strong interests in the health of others, and the progress of the pregnancy. Consent to the sharing of relevant information should be sought in the usual way. The ethical obligations to the pregnant woman and her child are no different to those owed to any woman and fetus for whom a duty of care has been accepted.

3:2.2 Patients considering self-insemination
General practitioners may be approached by women who are considering establishing a surrogate pregnancy by self-insemination. Doctors should encourage careful consideration of the issues and

implications and ensure that they have sufficient access to accurate information. The general practitioner will not necessarily be personally responsible for providing all the relevant information and counselling but must take all reasonable steps to see that the participants are aware of appropriate sources of advice, information, health testing and counselling.

3:2.3 Providing treatment services

Legal and ethical responsibilities increase considerably when health professionals are consulted in order to provide treatment services to establish a surrogate pregnancy. Such treatment services might involve insemination or more sophisticated reproductive technology such as in vitro fertilisation. By agreeing to examine and treat people in these circumstances, health professionals undertake an obligation to take proper account of the welfare of any child born or affected as a result of the treatment. This necessarily entails assessment of the circumstances into which a child will be born if treatment is successful and the impact the pregnancy may have on existing children of the surrogate or the intended parents, whether or not the pregnancy is carried to term.

3:3 Interests of the Child

The law requires those providing licensed treatment services (see section 2:2) to take into account the welfare of any child born or affected by the treatment before proceeding. The HFEA advises clinics to weigh the interests of the potential child with those of the other parties. From an ethical perspective, however, the BMA has consistently maintained that the interests of the potential child must be given precedence rather than simply figure as one of several factors.

When considering the interests of the potential child, the health care team should ensure that the combination of all foreseeable hazards, including any associated with the surrogacy, are not so great that they would preclude the likelihood of the child enjoying a satisfactory life. In practice, it is likely that the provision of treatment services is very rarely withheld on the grounds of the interests of the potential child, and some argue that even a difficult or miserable life is better than none. Whereas many individuals experiencing pain, abuse, neglect or other substantial disadvantages are nevertheless glad to have been born, most people regard it as axiomatic that it would be wrong knowingly to bring additional suffering into the world, even or especially to fulfil the desires of existing people.

Since there can be no unassailable guarantee which of the parties will eventually have care of a potential child, the clinician or health care team carrying out the assessment for assisted conception must take steps to verify that both the surrogate and the intended parents meet fundamental criteria for childcare. Physical disability should not prejudice assessment of the capacity of the various parties to undertake child rearing if sufficient necessary support is likely to be available. Anecdotal evidence and doctors' enquiries to the BMA, however, indicate that surrogacy arrangements are sometimes sought by women with a seriously life-threatening medical condition who would be unlikely to survive long beyond the birth of the child. While this might reflect an understandable stage of denial, health professionals must consider carefully the medical evidence, including the reliability of the diagnosis and discuss these sensitively with the intended parents. While health professionals should consider whether a child born under such an arrangement might be unacceptably disadvantaged by the potential loss of both the gestating mother (through the surrogacy arrangement) and the intended mother, the aims must be to reconcile the intended parents to the reality of their position and reach agreement in the weighing of likely risks and benefits. While surrogacy arrangements in such circumstances are not being ruled out altogether, each proposed pregnancy will require particularly careful and searching reflection. Further observations on this are made in section 5:1.2.

In itself, the fact of being born following a surrogacy arrangement is not sufficient disadvantage to the child to justify refusing the request of intended parents for assistance with conception. In many cases, there is some degree of uncertainty in the child's future, since the surrogacy arrangement cannot be enforced, but uncertainty is an inevitable facet of life. Although little evidence is available (see section 5:6), the risk of serious psychological harm to the child is considered low if open acknowledgement is made from an early stage in the child's life.

3:4 **Duties to Various Parties**

Part of the ethical complexity of surrogacy arises out of the competing interests of the various parties involved, to each of whom health professionals have a duty. Because two separate families are involved, care of the various parties is often shared between more than one general practitioner, community nurse and health visitor, possibly in areas of the country distant from each other. If the birth is planned to take place in hospital, antenatal care and labour involves other health professionals. A fertility clinic may be involved. In some cases, psychiatrists and other practitioners have also provided episodes of care to one of the parties and their reports may be relevant to the decisions made by other health professionals. At various stages there may be some overlapping professional and ethical responsibilities. It is important that all of the health professionals involved have a clear perspective as to which person has overall management of the pregnancy.

In this report, it is emphasised that the duties of confidentiality owed to each individual are not diminished by the fact that they have entered into a special agreement which allocates to others strong interests in each participant's health and lifestyle. It must also be recognised that, in the practice of health care no single ethical principle is absolute, and when foreseeable harm may be caused to others, including in the case of surrogacy a child or potential child, a justification for a breach of confidentiality may arise. In most cases, however, the parties concerned give their consent to relevant information being provided to those who need to know for the successful completion of the surrogacy arrangement.

In addition to the primary ethical obligation to consider the interests of the child, duties may also be owed by the same health care team to the intended parents, the surrogate and any existing children of each party. A balance must be maintained between the rights and needs of the various parties but health professionals have special obligations to the most vulnerable individuals, the children, who may have little or no opportunity to influence the decisions of the adults.

This section has attempted to identify which health professional is likely to have primary responsibility at each stage. These distinctions are not immutable and any health professional approached in connection with a request for advice or treatment as part of a surrogacy arrangement should consider whether he or she is the most appropriate person to provide it, or whether other expert sources of help are available.

3:4.1 Duties to intended parents and existing family

3:4.1.1 The initial enquiry

The general practitioner is often the first point of contact with the health system although some people may contact a fertility clinic directly. The doctor or other health professional receiving an initial enquiry should ensure that the intended parents have access to sufficient information to make a valid decision about proceeding. This should include information about:

- the alternative range of fertility treatment options (including the likelihood of success in their case);
- the availability of counselling (including counselling for involuntary childlessness), and the possibility of guilt, anxiety and uncertainty;
- the practical difficulties and financial costs of surrogacy (including the problem of finding a suitable woman willing to undertake the pregnancy);
- the medical and psychological risks of surrogacy (including risk of psychological problems for the child);
- the possibility of a multiple pregnancy if assisted reproduction techniques are used;
- the fact that, if a pregnancy is initiated, decisions as to the conduct or termination of the pregnancy will rest with the pregnant woman and not the intended parents even where the latter provided the sperm, eggs or embryos;
- the possibility of the surrogate mother engaging in activities which constitute a risk to the fetus;
- the possibility that the child may be born with a handicap;
- the possibility that the surrogate mother may wish to retain the child, and the unenforceability of any contractual arrangement; and
- the possibility of legal or other disputes between the parties.

The health professional receiving an initial enquiry may not have details of all these issues but must raise them as questions requiring thought.

If after having made reasonable efforts, the GP or other health professional cannot find counsellors or appropriate information, or if he or she has a conscientious objection to the whole procedure, patients should be referred to a colleague. If a GP has no objection in principle to surrogacy arrangements but considers that there are strong reasons against referring these particular individuals for advice and assessment (for example, if one of the intended parents suffers from a serious disease), these reasons should be fully and openly discussed with them. If, after discussion, they still wish to proceed the health professional should consider making a referral, subject to giving details of his or her reservations, having first sought the consent of the patients to such disclosure. In any case, efforts should be made to ensure that people do not feel abandoned if there is no likelihood of their plans proceeding. Putting people in touch with support groups or other therapists may help.

3:4.1.2 When a surrogacy arrangement is imminent

The clinician or health team must ensure that surrogacy is being considered only as a last resort, that both of the intended parents, where appropriate, are committed to having children and that the motivation of the intended parents is not based on any false assumption. The health of the intended parents should be compatible with the child being properly cared for and the clinician or health team must also consider, as far as can reasonably be anticipated, the effect of a surrogacy arrangement on any existing children of the intended parents or of the surrogate.

Even if other health professionals have already provided basic information and advice, it is important that immediately before proceeding the health team satisfy themselves that the intended parents know of:

- the risks involved;
- the availability of counselling;
- the availability of testing for infectious diseases such as HIV;
- the BMA's recommendations for encouraging informed openness between all parties involved;
- the importance of understanding the legal position; and

- the importance of ensuring that proper insurance cover has been arranged for the surrogate mother to benefit her family in the event of serious injury or death.

When a surrogacy arrangement is being initiated through treatment services provided by a licensed clinic, the clinic is likely to seek reports on the health of the intended parents as well as the surrogate. GPs, psychiatrists and specialists who have had care of the patients should seek to ensure that information relevant to the decision to proceed is made available, with the patient's consent. Exceptionally, if the gravity of the disclosure warrants and the patient refuses consent, a health professional may be justified in disclosing *limited relevant* information to the senior clinical member of the licensed centre.

3:4.1.3 *When a pregnancy is in progress*

Where a pregnancy has already been established, the principal obligations are similar to those for any other pregnancy and are owed primarily to the pregnant woman and her fetus. Special arrangements may be required to ensure that the intended parents may attend the antenatal preparations and birth and that the intended parents and surrogate mother receive home support from the health visitor or GP.

At this stage too, the clinician or health team responsible for the intended parents should ensure that, with the patients' consent, *relevant* information is made available to health professionals providing treatment services to the surrogate mother. In some exceptional cases, intended parents may refuse disclosure of information prejudicial to the fulfilment of the arrangement (for example, that they have criminal convictions for violence or child abuse or that they have a history of psychiatric ill-health). Because the predominant duty is owed to the potential child, health professionals who have such information and cannot persuade individuals to agree to disclosure, may decide, in exceptional circumstances, to breach confidentiality.

3:4.2 *Duties to the surrogate mother, her partner and family*

3:4.2.1 *The initial enquiry*

General practitioners may be approached by women interested in becoming a surrogate mother although some women take the first step by approaching a fertility clinic. The doctor or other health professional receiving an initial enquiry should ensure that the potential surrogate has access to sufficient information to make a valid decision, including information about:

- the practical difficulties, including those which arise from other people having strong views about how the pregnancy is conducted;
- the need to abstain from unprotected sexual intercourse during the months in which conception is attempted as part of a surrogacy arrangement;
- the medical risks associated with pregnancy, including those of postnatal depression and the psychological risks entailed in embarking on a process which many people might criticise;
- the risks associated with multiple pregnancy if assisted reproduction techniques are used;
- the possibilities of guilt, anxiety and a bereavement-like experience when the baby is given to the intended parents;
- the possibility that the child may be born with a handicap; and
- the availability of counselling.

The health professional initially approached may have reasons to consider that there are significant medical or psychological reasons why the woman should be advised against any pregnancy or a surrogacy arrangement. These should be discussed with her and referral to counsellors or other therapists arranged as appropriate.

3:4.2.2 When a surrogacy arrangement is imminent

Health professionals consulted by a woman who is planning pregnancy as a surrogate mother, by whatever means, should ensure that:

- her motivation is not based on false assumptions;
- her health is such that she will be capable of bearing a child without experiencing undue serious adverse health affects;
- she is aware of the options for testing for infectious diseases, such as HIV;
- she (and her partner) know of the risks involved, including the

special risks attached to IVF and other assisted reproduction, such as the risk of a multiple birth;

- she is aware of the potential for additional psychological burdens on other people if the pregnancy fails for any reason or has to be terminated;
- she has considered the psychological issues within her family, such as that other family members (including her existing children) may be distressed that she is willing to and does surrender the child or that her partner may resent her carrying a child for someone else; and
- she has considered the possibility that the child may be born with disabilities and that for that or other reasons the intended parents will not take the child.

Even if other health professionals have already provided basic information and advice, it is important that before proceeding the health team satisfy themselves that the surrogate mother (and her partner, where applicable) know of:

- the availability of counselling;
- the availability of testing for infectious diseases such as HIV;
- the BMA's recommendations for encouraging informed openness between all parties involved;
- the importance of understanding the legal position; and
- the importance of ensuring that proper insurance cover has been arranged to benefit her family in the event of serious injury or death.

3:4.2.3 When a pregnancy is in progress

When a pregnancy is already in progress, primary ethical responsibilities are to the pregnant woman and her fetus. Their well-being supersedes any agreement between the parties. Ideally, discussion should already have taken place about decision-making during the pregnancy. The BMA believes that, though full consultation is advisable at all stages, ultimately the responsibility for making such decisions lies with the pregnant woman, in consultation with health professionals. The latter must be aware that even when they provide care with conscientious attention to the woman's physical well-being, their own attitudes, especially if critical, can profoundly alter a woman's experience of pregnancy, birth or termination. It is important in this sensitive sphere as elsewhere, that once a decision has been made to provide care, it is provided sympathetically and non-judgmentally.

3:5 Coercion and Financial Pressures

Relations between individuals should be governed by respect for the needs and rights of others, whether they are autonomous adults or young children. Surrogacy is no different. It is vital that all those involved in a surrogacy arrangement do so freely and without coercion. Health professionals, social workers, lawyers or other professionals who become involved in surrogacy arrangements should be alert to the possibility of pressures being exerted. They must also consider whether the anxieties of any existing children or other family members of the surrogate mother are being addressed.

It is sometimes alleged that the general social differences and clearly differentiated economic status between those who contemplate surrogacy arrangements and women who undertake the pregnancy makes financial pressure inevitable. While most women who volunteer to undergo surrogate pregnancies appear to do so from altruistic motives, the possibility of obtaining financial assistance is also commonly a factor. (Surrogates are usually not "paid" but receive "reasonable expenses" which commonly range between £7-10,000.)

Evidence provided, by both intended parents and surrogates, for this report appears to indicate a generally high level of awareness and sensitivity in Britain about the hazards of promise-making and pressures being exerted. As far as can be judged anecdotally, this appears to be especially so when the parties are previously unknown to each other and begin to establish a basis of mutual trust without predetermined expectations. It may be that pressure is particularly likely when the surrogate is a relative or friend. In such cases, there may be a false assumption of mutual understanding which actually impedes open dissension so that the surrogate feels emotionally coerced into offering help. The possibility of subtle pressure brought by the intended parents or other family members may be unacknowledged or unperceived. Sometimes bringing repressed conflicts into the open may help the participants either to persuade others in a non-coercive way or accept that their own views will not prevail.

Health professionals should ensure that there are opportunities for the parties to be interviewed separately and for all to be aware of the possibility of unintended coercion. Adequate opportunities for counselling must be offered although uptake cannot be compelled. Those providing counselling should be ready to stress that obligations of kinship, although important, are not unlimited and that individuals are entitled to safeguard their own physical and emotional health.

Where health professionals consider that coercion is being applied or that the anxieties of vulnerable individuals, (including existing children) are being ignored, it is important that this possibility is addressed by all the parties. Health professionals should not simply absent themselves from the discussion even though it may appear in some cases that they can only make limited impact.

3:6 Testing for Infectious Diseases

In a surrogacy arrangement, it is advisable that the relevant parties consider being tested for infectious diseases such as HIV and hepatitis B. If treatment services are provided by a licensed clinic, relevant testing and counselling is arranged for the parties as appropriate. Where individuals are making their own arrangements, they should be aware of the opportunity for testing. Before any such test, individuals should be given the opportunity to be fully counselled about the implications of the results for themselves and their families. Health professionals consulted about a surrogacy arrangement should ensure that the counselling options available to each of the parties include testing and its implications.

3:7 The Relationship Between the Surrogate and the Intended Parents

In its 1990 report on surrogacy, the BMA considered that the desirability of anonymity between surrogate and intended parents was a matter of debate. Taking account of the limited studies and experience available in Britain at that time, the report recommended anonymity. This was based partly on reasoning about the likelihood of psychological distress for the surrogate who might find herself cosseted during the pregnancy but abruptly abandoned thereafter by intended parents anxious to establish a distance. Close relationships between the surrogate mother and the intended parents were also thought to give rise to potential uncertainty for the child and complex familial and relationship problems, which would be better avoided. Information about current practice does not appear to support these concerns.

The backdrop to this debate has altered substantially in the five years since the last report. British society has experienced changes in attitudes to infertility and the remedies available as well as significant modification in the range and type of family composition perceived as acceptable. Complex familial relationships are the norm for many people. They cannot be seen as *necessarily* damaging and the concomitant incentive to avoid them is reduced. People display greater awareness of their own health needs and what will help them flourish. Greater willingness to share information with children about their genetic background and the growing numbers of children born from the use of donated gametes, combined with an apparently increasing public acceptance of surrogacy means that decisions about anonymity are now made within a different framework. In addition, evidence from clinics offering IVF surrogacy and participants of surrogacy arrangements suggests that anonymity is no longer practical or desired by those undertaking the procedure. It has also been suggested that the required trust between the surrogate mother and the intended parents is best established though personal contact[16]. Such contact may continue after the child is relinquished. Also, many intended parents report that they plan to tell their child of the identity of the surrogate mother (see section 3:8 on openness and secrecy).

Meeting the other parties to a surrogacy arrangement may have the advantage of helping all those involved to form a positive and realistic image of one another. If a surrogate mother can hand the baby to the intended parents, this gives a positive emphasis to surrogacy as the gift of a treasured baby. The alternative situation, where the surrogate mother's baby vanishes and the intended parents' baby appears from nowhere, may be less satisfactory for all those involved. The legal changes recognised in the introduction of parental orders also makes any recommendation in favour of anonymity less practical.

Evidence currently indicates that contact between the parties *can* provide mutual support, although it cannot be assumed that this is a dependable feature of every arrangement. When relationships work well, they are reported as forming the basis of long-term friendships and may even play some compensatory role if the pregnancy fails to come to term. Open arrangements allow the intended parents to have involvement with the pregnancy, including being present at the birth of the baby. On the other hand, the expectation of achieving a fulfilling relationship between the parties can introduce additional problems and a sense of failure if it does not succeed. Some of the subtle pressures, discussed above, may be exacerbated if the intended parents would like further children with the same surrogate mother.

The BMA is conscious of the fact that many of those coming forward to give evidence may have been motivated to do so because their own experience has been a positive one and that a counterbalancing view is not so readily obtainable; people are perhaps reluctant to display the scars of damaging experiences. It considers, however, that it is perhaps now inappropriate for health professionals to attempt to lay down firm rules on a matter which is increasingly perceived as a social issue, without strong evidence of a health detriment.

On balance, the conclusion of this report is that it must be for individuals to consider the matter carefully and make their own decisions about the type of relationship they think appropriate. On a practical level, while some people report benefits arising from maintaining contact between the parties after the birth, this will not suit everybody. For some surrogates, continuing contact may ease the difficulties in surrendering the child but for others it may have the opposite effect. It is important to stress, therefore, that the nature and degree of contact depends on the particularities of each case, specifically the wishes and preferences of those directly involved.

3:8 Openness and Secrecy

Whilst anonymity is currently practised in donor insemination, and is common in adoption, it is no longer regarded as desirable by everyone. It appears that secrecy is sometimes seen by one parent as a means of protecting the sensitivity and self-esteem of the other. This has traditionally been the case in instances of male infertility which has been underestimated for social reasons and deliberately hidden. Better public awareness of the frequency of male infertility and of the difference between fertility and sexuality has permitted more informed discussion. If the parties have opportunities to discuss their feelings, it may be that the perceived need to protect such sensitivities will diminish.

There is now growing social recognition of the potential benefits of openness with children born following all forms of assisted conception. Without pressuring them to make decisions with which they feel profoundly uncomfortable, health professionals should try to ensure that the intended parents are aware of the problems that may arise when secrets are kept between members of families. If an application is made for a parental order, "dual registration" of the birth occurs and a person may, on reaching 18, have access to the original birth certificate, identifying the surrogate mother. Unexpected and unplanned disclosure may damage relationships.

Experience from adoption shows that it is beneficial to be open and explicit at an early age, and similar advice should be given in surrogacy cases, coupled with practical assistance to parents in developing the skills necessary for such honesty and openness. It is important that intended parents are aware that, as with adoption, children's understanding of surrogacy may not proceed in a gradual way. The acceptance which characterises the early years of childhood will probably change between 6 and 8 years of age to a more complex attitude characterised by worry, questioning, withdrawal and acting out of, for example, aggressive behaviour. At this stage the child will be able to acknowledge the loss involved in surrogacy, and may begin to explore the motives of the adults involved. Children's behaviour may therefore appear to undergo a sudden change, becoming undesirable or unacceptable to the parents. With partial surrogacy, parents may attribute such behaviour to the surrogate mother's genetic inheritance. Awareness of the reason for this type of behaviour is therefore important.

If partial surrogacy is used, there may sometimes be medical reasons making it advisable for the child to be aware of his or her genetic origins. The BMA, however, tends to the view that the importance of these is often exaggerated. In making diagnoses or recommendations for later treatment, no health professional relies on the assumption that the social parents are necessarily the genetic progenitors of the child. Increasingly sophisticated genetic screening places reliance on testing individuals rather than gaining information at second hand from other (real or supposed) family members. However, the demand for genetic screening for employment and insurance purposes can only increase and these developments are likely to make long-term secrecy within families impracticable. This issue is considered further in chapter 5.

3:9 Ethics Committees

Many fertility clinics have ethics committees to consider difficult ethical dilemmas which arise in connection with the provision of fertility services. Some clinics submit every potential case of surrogacy for consideration and some committees use a set of background principles as a framework for assessing the merits of each case. The advantage of access to an ethics committee is that it offers clinicians an independent multi-disciplinary perspective[17]. The BMA considers it helpful to have access to such advice, especially in difficult cases.

4 Medical Aspects of Surrogacy

There are few differences in purely clinical terms between the problems which are likely to occur in a surrogate pregnancy and any other pregnancy, although there is the potential for psychological problems (which are discussed in chapter 5) and the difficulties related to the increased possibility of a multiple pregnancy if assisted reproduction techniques are used. With surrogacy, however, the pregnant woman undertakes the risks for the benefit of another person rather than primarily for herself. It is, therefore, particularly important that health professionals providing treatment services to establish the pregnancy ensure that the surrogate is aware of any problems that could arise. Ideally the potential surrogate mother should have successfully carried a previous pregnancy to term and therefore be aware of conditions associated with pregnancy especially her own experiences and emotions. The health team providing the treatment services also has a moral responsibility to consider the potential surrogate mother's partner and family and the intended parents. In view of the nature of the procedures involved and the need for follow up of the surrogate throughout and after the pregnancy, health professionals involved with initiating a surrogate pregnancy should be aware that this may represent a long-term commitment. Before providing treatment services to establish a surrogate pregnancy, consideration should be given to the medical and psychological needs of those participating in the arrangement. This chapter addresses some of the main medical issues which need to be addressed.

4:1 Health of Intended Parents

One fundamental safeguard for the well-being of a future child is the medical assessment of all the parties to the surrogacy arrangement. If the intended parents are donating gametes, medical examination should include screening for genetically transmissible conditions as well as the presence of any infection which could be passed to the surrogate mother. It is vital that intended parents give consideration to this, particularly if the surrogate is planning self-insemination without medical involvement.

Since surrogacy should only be regarded as a solution of last resort, medical staff should satisfy themselves, before becoming involved with a surrogacy arrangement, that the intended parents have tried all other reasonable options.

Health professionals providing treatment services to establish a surrogate pregnancy must be aware of any adverse health problems which could affect the intended parents' ability to raise the child, before agreeing to assist with the arrangement. In rare cases, where one partner has a condition which is likely to be fatal or severely disabling, the effect of that on a potential child has to be carefully considered. In most cases health professionals would be very reluctant to assist in establishing a pregnancy and bringing a child into existence if there is a significant likelihood of one or both of its parents dying whilst the child is very young.

If the health professional consulted about the surrogacy arrangement is not the general practitioner of the intended parents, it is recommended that, with their consent, advice is sought from their GP, about any factors which might be relevant to the treatment. The GP might have information which is important to the overall assessment of the interests of the patients and the potential child. Again in rare cases, this might, for example, be information about previous child abuse or neglect. Some health professionals who are not providing treatment services or advising on surrogacy may, nonetheless, be aware that a person is considering surrogacy. In such cases, the practitioner should seek to persuade them to share relevant information with the medical team providing the treatment services. If such information highlights an *exceptional* risk to any of the parties involved, including the potential child, the person should be informed that the practitioner might consider it imperative to disclose such information without their consent. In such cases, the person should first be advised of this intention and be given the opportunity to divulge the relevant information, or to discuss further the implications of disclosure. Where a health professional has significant, well-grounded concerns about the ability of the couple to bring up a child, for whatever reason, and a medical team is not involved with the arrangement, the practitioner should advise the couple to see a counsellor before proceeding. If the couple decide to proceed without counselling and against the practitioner's advice, they cannot simply be abandoned and medical care should still be offered.

4:2 Health of the Surrogate Mother

Medical assessment of the potential surrogate mother is particularly important both regarding the possibility of inadvertently transmitting genetic disorders if her own gametes are used and in relation to her ability to undergo a pregnancy with minimum risk to her own health. If there are any medical problems which could lead to serious complications with the pregnancy, or put the woman at risk, this must be seriously considered and discussed with her. As maternal morbidity and mortality are higher in a first pregnancy, it is strongly recommended that the surrogate mother should have borne at least one child previously and preferably have completed her own family. Having experienced pregnancy prior to the surrogacy arrangement she can also consider aspects of the agreement from a position of knowledge. As mentioned in section 5:2.2, for example, the risk of postnatal depression may be reduced for a surrogate mother who already has children of her own. Other factors relating to the more general health of the surrogate mother should also be considered. Evidence of heavy smoking, drinking or substance abuse should give cause for concern. As with the intended parents, if the doctor involved is not the surrogate mother's general practitioner, enquiries should be made of the GP, with the woman's consent, seeking relevant information. Similarly, any other practitioner with relevant information should seek to persuade the intending surrogate mother to share that information with those providing the treatment services or with a counsellor.

4:3 Health Risks of Surrogacy

With surrogacy using IVF, the sperm or embryos are quarantined whilst repeated tests are undertaken on the intended parents (or other donors) to screen for HIV, hepatitis and other infections or genetic disorders. If untested sperm or eggs are used the surrogate is at risk of infection, with medical and possible legal repercussions (see section 2:8). If self-insemination is to be used, health professionals have a duty to inform the surrogate mother, and the intended parents, of the risk of infection and to encourage them to seek testing to minimise the risks.

Although using IVF cuts down the risk of infection by using quarantined sperm or embryos, it is not itself without risks. The intended mother, if her eggs are to be used, is usually given drugs to stimulate her ovaries so that more than one egg is produced. There are known side-effects to the use of these drugs, the most common of which is ovarian hyperstimulation syndrome (OHSS). This is usually very mild but in about 1% of cases can be serious and require hospitalisation. The eggs are usually collected using an ultrasound guided needle which may be painful. The surrogate mother undergoes tests and takes drugs to prepare her for the embryos which are to be implanted and to synchronise her menstrual cycle (if the embryos are not to be cryopreserved). If more than one embryo is replaced, in IVF surrogacy, the risk of multiple pregnancy increases and, with standard IVF in 1993, the multiple pregnancy rate increased from 21.5% to 31.2% with the increase from two to three embryos[18]. With the replacement of three embryos there is also a much higher chance of a triplet or higher order multiple pregnancy with the associated risks for both mother and babies. In view of the high risk of multiple pregnancy with IVF, careful consideration should be given to the number of embryos to be replaced and some health professionals recommend that no more than two embryos are replaced. In all cases of IVF surrogacy, the decision about the number of embryos to be replaced, subject to the maximum specified by the HFEA, should rest with the surrogate mother in conjunction with the relevant health professionals.

Surrogate pregnancies are no more likely to have adverse effects on the woman's physical health than any other pregnancy (apart from risks associated with multiple pregnancy). However, the surrogate should be made aware of these usual risks of pregnancy. In rare cases, estimated to be around 10 in 100,000, pregnancy can result in maternal death[19]. In view of this small risk, the intended parents should be strongly encouraged to purchase insurance to benefit the surrogate's family in case of serious injury or death. There are other less dramatic, but more frequent, health risks with pregnancy. Problems may arise during the pregnancy or in the period after the birth such as: gestational diabetes, pre-eclampsia, urinary-tract infections, haemorrhage, stress incontinence (19% of women in one study[20]), painful intercourse (20% in the same study) and haemorrhoids. A 1993 study[21] found that 85% of women had at least one health problem in the immediate post-partum period, whilst in hospital, and 87% had at least one problem at home. Doctors providing treatment services or giving advice about surrogacy have a duty to ensure that the potential surrogate mother is aware of, and has understood, these risks.

The psychological aspects of surrogacy are discussed in chapter 5.

4:4 Decision-making During Pregnancy

During the pregnancy itself a number of decisions need to be taken, some of which require a balance to be reached between the well-being of the woman and the fetus. Whilst, ideally, a joint decision can be reached between the surrogate mother and the intended parents, there may be times when their views are in conflict. It is important that before the surrogacy arrangement proceeds everyone involved is clear and understands that the surrogate mother, in conjunction with the health professionals, will make the final decision. Decisions during pregnancy might include various tests to be undertaken such as ultrasound, blood, HIV, hepatitis B and inherited disorders. Tests such as amniocentesis and Chorion Villus Sampling (CVS) introduce risks for the woman and for the fetus. Intended mothers tend to be older than the norm, partly because they may have been through repeated tests and possibly treatment for infertility. If the intended mother's eggs are used there might be an increased risk of chromosomal abnormality. It is likely, therefore, that the proportion of pregnancies where tests such as amniocentesis are indicated will be higher than average. It must also be discussed and clarified before a pregnancy is established who will decide how to proceed if a severe abnormality is detected.

The BMA's view is that this decision must rest with the carrying mother but that the options should be discussed between the parties *before the arrangement is made*. If the intended parents feel they would be unable to look after a child with a severe handicap and the surrogate mother is opposed to termination, the parties need to decide how the situation would be managed and, if agreement cannot be reached, whether the surrogacy arrangement should proceed. Cases may occur where one party has a change of mind when the situation arises. Discussing the matter in advance attempts to ensure that the likelihood of this happening is minimised.

4:5 Decisions about Method of Delivery

Another issue which needs to be discussed in advance is the preferred method of delivery. It is important for all concerned to know if, for example, the surrogate mother wishes to give birth in water or if the intended parents are totally opposed to the use of drugs during delivery. Conflicts may arise between the best interests of the surrogate mother and those of the baby. If the baby is in breach position, for example, a choice has to be made about whether to attempt to turn the baby around manually, to carry out a vaginal breach delivery or to undertake a caesarian, which may be better for the baby but has implications for the woman. Decisions might have to be made about whether to induce the pregnancy; whether to give drugs such as pethidine, which eases the pain for the woman but can cause respiratory suppression in the newborn baby; or an epidural, which will reduce pain but can prolong labour. In the latter stages of labour, decisions might need to be made about, for example, whether to have a forceps delivery or ventouse extraction. The BMA believes that decisions about delivery should be made by the surrogate mother, together with the health professionals. But these issues should be addressed prior to concluding the arrangement.

Other decisions need to be taken during and immediately after the delivery about which parents would normally be consulted, particularly in the case of a preterm delivery. Ideally, a joint decision could be reached but, as the parental orders provision allows a six week period for the surrogate mother to reflect on her decision to surrender the child, she should also have the right to make decisions about the child immediately after delivery. In the days after the delivery, provided the child has been given to the intended parents, responsibilities for decision-making should pass to them.

4:6 Breast Milk

In surrogacy arrangements, the baby is very rarely breast fed. It is important for those involved to recognise that this could lead to disadvantages for the child, particularly if the baby is born preterm. There are, of course, many babies who are not breast fed and are perfectly healthy. If the intended parents wish to feed their baby breast milk, there are some options open to them. It is possible, for example, for the intended mother to induce breast milk, although this is rarely very successful and can add to her distress. Alternatively, the surrogate mother could provide breast milk although again this happens very rarely. From a practical point of view it is time consuming and will prolong the effects of the labour for her when she might prefer to get back to her usual lifestyle as soon as possible after the delivery. Some of the potential consequences of breast feeding are discussed further in section 5:4.1. Advice may be sought from health professionals on the feasibility of the various options.

4:7 Support for the Surrogate Mother

A pregnant woman is entitled to appropriate standards of medical care irrespective of the circumstances of her pregnancy. Surrogacy is no reason for a different approach. The usual post-delivery health follow up should be offered and arrangements for additional emotional support considered when the baby is given to the intended parents. In some circumstances it might be appropriate to offer counselling to the surrogate mother (therapeutic counselling is discussed in section 6:4.4).

4:8 Support for the Intended Parents

Once the baby has been given to the intended parents, they should be offered the same support services as any other family with a newborn baby. Arrangements should be made for a midwife and health visitor to visit the family and for the usual health checks to be carried out on the baby. In the event of the surrogate mother deciding to keep the child, emotional support should be available to the intended parents and consideration given to the possibility of a referral for professional counselling (again discussed in section 6:4.4).

5 Psychological Aspects of Surrogacy

Although there is now a substantial body of literature on the psychological and social aspects of infertility and its treatment, it is only very recently that surrogacy has been the focus of research. What information is available tends to come from small-scale studies, and it is not known to what extent it is possible to generalise from these to the experience of those involved in surrogacy procedures. It is particularly important to note that the psychological and social implications of surrogacy are likely to change should surrogacy become more widespread.

It is now becoming recognised that there is much more variation in family structure and routes to parenthood than previously understood. Whilst surrogate mothers and intended parents are faced with many difficult tasks, from a psychological point of view surrogacy does not appear to pose greater problems than those tolerated for conventional and assisted reproduction parenting[22]. This means that in considering the psychological significance of surrogacy, evidence can be drawn from relevant areas, including studies of the psychological aspects of adoption, gamete donation and other reproductive techniques. All of these hold an important message for surrogacy: children *can and do* grow up happily with adults who are not their biological or genetic parents.

5:1 Motivations

5:1.1 Surrogate mothers

Whilst there is increasing interest in the characteristics of surrogate mothers, few studies have made more than a superficial examination of their motivations. What information there is suggests that whilst financial gain may be the only motive for some, women usually decide to become surrogate mothers for a number of reasons[23-29]. Their desire to help may be characterised by some or all of the following factors:

- financial need, often for a particular purpose (in one study, 40% of mothers gave this as the main reason);
- a high value placed on children and parenthood, together with a feeling that they are fortunate to be mothers;
- great sympathy with childless people;
- easy and enjoyable experiences of pregnancy and childbirth and a desire to re-experience these without the responsibility of rearing the child, or in the absence of the resources to support one;
- a wish for enhanced self-esteem or self-worth to be gained from helping others;
- health problems which surrogacy may overcome (for example, to "treat" endometriosis); or
- an attempt to resolve feelings associated with previous reproductive losses (for example, termination of pregnancy or giving up a child for adoption).

Some surrogacy arrangements are made within families, such as with a sister or mother, or with friends. Motivations under such circumstances are difficult to determine, as they may involve some sense of duty or responsibility, and may sometimes be the result of coercion.

5:1.2 Intended parents

Although intended parents' motivations for parenthood have not been studied, there is no reason to suppose that they are different from the majority of people. Indeed, a willingness to consider surrogacy as a method of having children suggests that their desire for parenthood is very strong, and a strong desire for parenthood appears to be more important for good family functioning than genetic relationships.

There are many reasons why people wish to have children. These include acceptance as a responsible and mature member of the community which parenthood usually confers, the need to give and receive affection, the desire for stimulation and interest in life which having children can bestow, and the wish to have someone carrying on for oneself after one's death. This last motivation may be intensified in those who are involuntarily childless and have a terminal or life-threatening illness: the prospect of a child may mean that something of themselves can be kept alive. People already experiencing the stresses of infertility and of terminal illness may be quite reasonably preoccupied with their own needs and therefore find it difficult to consider the welfare of a child, especially one not yet conceived. Health professionals need to be satisfied that the welfare of the child will not be jeopardised. It is therefore essential in these circumstances that all who are involved give particular consideration to what might happen to the child in the event of the parent's death, and the possible implications for a child who has been relinquished by one parent and then faces the loss of another. Such cases will require clear articulation of the possible detriments as well as an account of the benefits, and especially sensitive consideration.

5:2 Implications for the Surrogate Mother

5:2.1 Attachment to the fetus and baby

Although feelings of attachment to the fetus generally increase over the course of a pregnancy, it is normal for a woman's feelings to fluctuate. Prenatal feelings of attachment to the fetus have been found to be strongly related to feelings about the baby after the delivery. Thus a surrogate mother who develops strong attachment during pregnancy is likely to find it particularly difficult to relinquish the child. Whilst surrogate mothers appear to be more detached from their fetus than is usual, they may come to love the baby by the ninth month[30]. Such an attachment is advantageous in that it is likely to discourage the woman from behaving in a way that would otherwise risk her health and that of the fetus. However, a surrogate mother's relationship with the child both during pregnancy and afterwards may well be very ambivalent. She might start by feeling good about the gesture she is making to the couple, but gradually experience a sense of conflict, apprehension or even guilt. These feelings could, at the time of the birth, result in her deciding to keep the child, despite entailing that she has to bring up a child she had not planned to keep. Even if she does relinquish the child, feelings of pain, anger and guilt might persist for a very long time, and be coupled with fears that the child was not being properly loved and cared for.

It is sometimes suggested that full surrogacy is preferable to partial surrogacy, because the surrogate will not have made a genetic contribution in the former case and so may feel less of a sense of loss

45

on parting with the child. However, as people vary in their feelings about the importance of genetic relationships, this may not hold for all surrogate mothers. Also important may be the consideration that if the baby is genetically related to the surrogate mother, it may remind her of her own children and therefore make it harder for her to relinquish.

While the BMA acknowledges that there is very little systematic information on the experience of surrogacy, what little there is suggests that only a small proportion of surrogate mothers go so far as to retain the child[31]. It is certainly a smaller proportion than those mothers who plan to release their child for adoption but change their mind when the baby is born.

5:2.2 Postnatal psychological reactions
The surrogate mother should be aware of the risk of postnatal depression, as well as the fact that experience of postnatal depression carries a risk of relapse with subsequent babies.

Women's risk of depressive illness is substantially increased after childbirth: rates of depression any time in the first year after delivery are in the order of 10-20%. The exact cause is undetermined, but it is not solely the result of hormonal influences. Vulnerability factors specific to postnatal depression include previous psychiatric history, lack of employment, housing problems, poor marital relations, lack of social and emotional support and little previous contact with babies. Women experiencing postnatal depression commonly feel inadequate, angry, helpless or hopeless. Experiences of depressed mood are likely to be exacerbated by economic privation, disturbed sleep and physical exhaustion. In cases of mild depression, simply allowing women to talk about their experience and feelings can be valuable in alleviating depression.

There are no data on the incidence of postnatal depression in surrogate mothers. Precipitating factors suggest that the risk of depression may be reduced for surrogate mothers who already have children of their own and who have partners able to provide support. However, given that many psychological factors thought to be important in the development of such depression relate to the woman's experience with her baby (for example, inability to cope, social isolation), it might be expected that surrogate mothers would be *less* vulnerable to postnatal depression. On the other hand, the surrogate mother has chosen to relinquish the baby, and therefore may experience the sort of emotional distress normally associated with perinatal loss. A small study of surrogate mothers found that 75% of women reported moderate or severe depression "which included uncontrollable sobbing, sleep dysfunction, aching arms and difficulty interacting with other newborns" which lasted from 2 to 6 weeks[30]. In one case the woman had to be hospitalised.

Surrogate mothers who suffer from postnatal depression may require less practical support than mothers who have a baby to deal with, but their need for psychological support is likely to be just as great. If depression persists, treatment or referral to a psychiatrist should be considered, particularly if the surrogate has children of her own.

5:3 Implications for the Surrogate Mother's Family

There are additional implications for the surrogate's partner, her existing children and her parents.

It is important that the surrogate mother's partner is able to give his (or perhaps exceptionally her) full support for the woman's decision to act as a surrogate mother. Whilst she is trying to become pregnant, heterosexual couples will need to refrain from unprotected intercourse, which could strain their relationship. Partners will need to provide emotional support during the pregnancy and after parting with the child, when they themselves may experience conflicts about losing the baby their partner has carried. In the event of the mother deciding to keep the baby, although she may experience guilt and other emotions associated with the failure to keep to her agreement, she will clearly want the baby. However, her partner may find it difficult to accept a child conceived from another man[22]. In supporting the surrogate mother her partner should be advised that he may, under the provisions of the Human Fertilisation and Embryology Act 1990 be regarded *in law* as the father of the child (see section 2:4). There may therefore be some risk of psychological problems for the surrogate mother's partner. In general, however, the surrogate mother's need for support makes it desirable that she has a partner rather than being without one.

Other children of the surrogate mother need to be informed of what is happening and, unless very well supported at the time of birth, may be distressed by the disappearance of a baby. If the mother achieves some detachment from the pregnancy and baby, children may find this confusing and may worry that they could be rejected and "discarded" in a similar way. In addition, the surrogate mother's parents may experience difficulty in understanding their daughter's decision and find it hard to relinquish a relationship with a baby who might otherwise have been their grandchild.

It is important that those involved recognise that close family and friends of the surrogate mother are likely to have mixed feelings about what is happening, and might be pressed to explain the arrangement to the outside world.

5:4 Implications for the Intended Parents

In making the decision to proceed with surrogacy, the intended parents face a great deal of uncertainty. They might feel guilt about the arrangement, coupled with a worry that, however rare in practice, the child will not be relinquished. They may be concerned with uncertainty about the adoption or parental orders process. They might worry about their reaction to the child being born handicapped; and, with partial surrogacy, they may harbour doubts that the child's parentage is as claimed. They might also fear that information about the arrangement will fall into the wrong hands. They may even come to regard the child not as a release from their childlessness, but as a continuing reminder of their inability to produce a child without help.

5:4.1 Attachment to the fetus or baby

Some intended parents may be concerned that they will not be able to accept the child as their own. If partial surrogacy is used, the woman, in particular, might be concerned that she will not become attached to the child, and that she will find it difficult to accept the biological child of her partner and another woman. However, it is clear that successful attachment relationships form between parents and children even when parents have no genetic relationship with the child and are not present immediately after delivery. Attachment is not something that is only formed during a critical period after delivery, but develops gradually over a period of time. The intended parents have the advantage over adoptive parents of having nine months in which to prepare for the baby's appearance.

The importance of early interactions and continuity of parenting should not, however, be underestimated. Babies learn very fast: for example, within a few days of birth they have learned the particular way in which they are held when fed, and can anticipate the breast or bottle as soon as they are held in this way. They quickly learn to distinguish their mother's face from another's and, if breast fed, to recognise the smell of her milk. Whenever a baby is transferred to a different mother or parents, relationships will be disrupted, and the baby is likely to share its distress with its new parents. These effects are probably transient, but all attempts should be made to reduce the distress caused to the baby, in view of its dependence on adults[22]. Thus, it is likely to be beneficial for the baby to establish contact with the intended parents as soon as possible after delivery.

Breast feeding has advantages for the baby's physical health, but the relationship between breast feeding and the development of attachment between mother and baby is not clear. Whilst there is some suggestion that breast feeding immediately after delivery leads to stronger bonding, this does not necessarily imply that bonding will occur if the surrogate mother wishes to feed the child. The intended mother should be aware that it may be possible for her to establish breast feeding with the baby.

5:4.2 Psychological reactions

An intended mother who lacks experience with babies may have to deal with the additional belief that the "natural" mother could have cared for the baby better than she is able to do. Moreover, psychosocial factors implicated in postnatal depression (lack of social and emotional support, social isolation) may equally apply to women who have to care for babies after adoption or surrogacy. An intended mother may have a small risk of developing depression after receiving the child. It has been estimated that about 1 in 2000 women experience post-adoptive depression.

Intended parents should be aware that it is not unusual for marital satisfaction to decline in some respects after the birth of a baby. Should marital problems be experienced, this should not necessarily be attributed to the surrogacy arrangement.

5:4.3 *Anonymity and telling the child*

One question which all intended parents have to deal with is whether to tell their child of his or her origins. Most people who choose surrogacy report that they have decided to explain the circumstances of the conception and birth to their child[23]. If parents decide not to tell, they face a number of difficulties. Surrogacy is thought to be difficult to conceal from others, and if other people know about the arrangement, then the child may find out from them (whether deliberately or inadvertently). The experience of learning in this way, and the discovery of deception by his or her parents may be very distressing for a child. Such an experience may have long-term implications for the parent-child relationship. Even if a child does not discover in this way, a lack of openness may mean that the parents have difficulty in communicating with their child on related topics - sex, contraception, fertility, genetic and family relationships, and family health problems. Such communication difficulties may lead the child to suspect that he or she is unusual, but discourage the child from trying to discuss these issues with his or her parents. Thus, in addition to general reasons for encouraging honesty with children, it may not be feasible, or in the child's long-term interests, for the truth to be withheld. The intended parents should also be aware that at 18 a person has a legal right to discover the identity of his or her surrogate mother.

Adoptive parents can use information about their child's birth mother to aid the process of telling the child. Parents with children conceived by donor insemination comment on the difficulty of talking in the absence of any information about the genetic father. An information profile on the surrogate mother might, therefore, be helpful in enabling parents to tell their child of her or his origins. Keeping the surrogate mother informed of the child's progress via reports may both ease any grief and provide recognition of her help. The BMA has been told by one of the self-help surrogacy support groups that arrangements which they foster on a non-commercial basis are often undertaken with open contact between all the parties, before and after birth, with a positive outcome for all[32]. However, there has been no scientific examination of the psychological implications of anonymity or personal contact for parents or children involved in surrogacy arrangements. What is important, therefore, is that the surrogate mother and intended parents agree on a level of contact which they feel is appropriate for them.

5:5 Implications for the Intended Parents' Family

Intended parents need to be aware of the possible implications for other members of their family. This might include existing children, who need careful preparation for the arrival of the baby. It is also possible that surrogacy may cause difficulties for grandparents, who may treat this grandchild differently.

5:6 Implications for the Child

There is almost no research into the effects of surrogacy on the resulting children. However, from a psychological point of view, there are great similarities between surrogacy and adoption arrangements. The child is the one person in a surrogacy arrangement who has no choice in the matter. It is therefore essential that all decisions taken about the advisability of proceeding are viewed from the perspective of the child's best interests - even, if necessary, at the expense of the interests of the adult parties.

5:6.1 The fetus and the baby

Concern has been expressed that a surrogate mother's detachment from her fetus and baby might lead her to risk the fetus's or the baby's health. However, there is no evidence to suggest that this occurs. Whilst breast feeding has advantages for the baby's well-being, it is very rare that the surrogate mother wishes to breast feed. Clearly, this is a matter for her to decide in consultation with the intended parents and in the light of her experience of feeding other children. If she has always fed her children with bottle milk, following the birth of a baby intended for other parents is probably not the time to initiate breast feeding. It may be less disruptive for the baby to be fed by the intended mother or parents from the start.

5:6.2 The child

It has been suggested that a child born through surrogacy may feel anxiety about being different from others, may feel ashamed, may wish to know more but be unwilling to ask for fear of distressing his or her parents, and may feel that his or her parents' expectations are unrealistic. Children's anxieties can often be reduced by parents who are willing to acknowledge the difference between their family and others (rather than rejecting the difference), without suggesting

51

that "difference" implies "deficiency". Parents who reject the difference between their family and others may make it difficult for children to ask questions about their origins and birth mother.

Particular concern has been expressed about the effects on a child of having been relinquished by a parent; having been told, honestly and openly, that it was born following a surrogacy arrangement, the fear is that a child might experience a sense of rejection based upon the fact that a woman was prepared to give up her child at birth. However, children who are born following surrogacy can be reassured that their existence is entirely due to the strong desire of their parents to have a child.

In addition, it has been proposed that the child may face a loss of status, and may be stigmatised, because he or she is different from other children. However, the notion that children might be taunted or rejected by their peers does not appear to be true for other "different" families (for example, children of lesbian parents). More positively, it has been suggested that people conceived via a surrogacy arrangement may in fact be proud of their parents' courage and grateful to their parents for their existence.

6 Counselling

6:1 Who Needs Counselling?

For some people, the apparent solution offered by surrogacy results in bitter disappointment, confusion or depression. This may happen if, for example, pregnancies repeatedly fail, the genetic child of the intended parents is withheld by the surrogate or the child is born severely disabled. Participation, even in a straightforward surrogacy arrangement, can be complex and stressful. Chapter 5 analysed the range of psychological reactions which may occur in people associated with a surrogacy arrangement and drew attention to the way in which discussion and support can be helpful in enabling people to identify key difficulties.

The stresses are not necessarily restricted to the main participants in a surrogacy arrangement but can affect those who appear to be on the periphery, such as the family or relatives of the surrogate mother or those of the intended parents. It is essential that all have ample opportunity to make their views known and to give careful consideration in advance to the potential medical, social and legal issues both for themselves and for other people towards whom they may have some responsibility. The partner and existing children of the surrogate should not be overlooked when access to counselling is discussed. Their reactions at relinquishing the child may be quite different to how they feel during the pregnancy. For them there may be difficulties either in accepting the pregnancy or parting with a child. In most cases of partial surrogacy that child will be a half-sibling of the existing children with all the implications of shared family resemblances and genetic heritage.

Although offering to undertake surrogacy for an infertile couple might appear to be an uncomplicated altruistic act, it is not an easy course of action and all parties must be clear about the implications of their decision before proceeding. A potential surrogate mother must consider carefully her likely emotional reactions to the developing fetus, the possibility of miscarriage or termination and the effect of parting with the child if the pregnancy is successful. There may be a risk of postnatal depression.

The intended mother may worry about her potential ability to bond with a child carried by another woman or fear that the surrogate mother will decide to keep the child. All of these issues can be aired in counselling. While access to appropriate counselling should not be seen as a panacea for all the anxieties which accompany the uncertainties of fertility treatments generally and surrogacy in particular, specially trained and knowledgeable counsellors can provide reassurance about the commonality of the varied emotions experienced by people in this situation.

The Human Fertilisation and Embryology Act 1990 section 13(6) provides that people considering assisted conception through a licensed centre be given "a suitable opportunity to receive proper counselling about the implications of taking the proposed steps"[33]. Individuals consulting health professionals in such centres with regard to a surrogate pregnancy must be offered such counselling before any medical procedures are undertaken. The report of the King's Fund Counselling Committee[34] suggests that the legal requirement to offer counselling is reinforced by the further legal obligation for health professionals to take account of the welfare of any child who may be born, and other children who might be affected by the birth. The BMA strongly recommends that people considering surrogacy be actively encouraged to take advantage of counselling in order to satisfy themselves that they have fully considered the issues and their implications.

Counselling should not be seen either as an optional luxury or as indicative of some deficiency in the participants of the arrangement but as an integral element of surrogacy arrangements. Counselling might also continue during and after the pregnancy, rather than be restricted to the period before the arrangement is established. Continuing availability of counselling might be particularly important for surrogate mothers, some of whom experience bereavement-like emotions after parting with the child, or who may have to deal with sentiments of failure or guilt if the pregnancy miscarries. Counselling is also likely to be valuable after the child is born for intended parents considering how and when to inform the child of his or her origins. The availability of counselling should be continuous rather than limited to one brief, specific stage of the arrangement, and in section 6:4 the different types of counselling, which may at some stage be appropriate, are clarified.

6:2 Aims of Counselling

Often, when counselling is discussed in the context of surrogacy, it is presumed that its main purpose is to ease the participants through the uncertainties and possible disappointments of the attempts at achieving pregnancy and carrying it to term. This is indubitably one of the main purposes. In the BMA's view, however, in addition to helping those involved with surrogacy to think through the emotional and practical issues of proceeding, counselling may help some infertile people to come to terms with their childlessness. This should also be seen as a successful outcome.

6:3 Counselling About Childlessness

Increasing recognition is given to the many subtle means by which individuals are pressurised to meet certain social norms. The education system, the media, popular culture or simply the expectations of family and friends influence people in their assessment of what is necessary for them to achieve personal satisfaction. Feminist writers and commentators in particular have drawn attention to the pressures on women to have children and to the social stigma still attached to those who cannot or who freely choose not to do so. People who seek to remedy their childlessness through surrogacy have almost invariably thought deeply about it as well as having explored all other feasible options. In some cases, however, the imperative to exhaust every avenue can take on a momentum of its own and people cannot give up the pursuit until they have satisfied themselves that for them surrogacy does not offer a realistic way forward. Counselling may assist in identifying this stage in the process.

Although it evidently succeeds for some people, surrogacy is inappropriate for others. The main aim of offering counselling should be to assist individuals and couples to accept their situation. At several points in this report, attention has been drawn to the exceptional cases where intended parents place all their hopes on achieving their own genetic child through surrogacy, almost as a distraction from dealing with the diagnosis of a life-threatening illness in themselves or their partner, or other life difficulties. Such cases of a person's denial of the implications of his or her condition are mentioned because they form a small but persistent core of ethical enquiries to the BMA from doctors. The ethical responsibilities discussed in chapter 3 clarify that such patients need considerable support and should not be abandoned. Therapeutic counselling, discussed in section 6:4.4, may provide one facet of that support.

6:4 Surrogacy Counselling

The principal aims of counselling are discussed in some detail in the King's Fund report on the counselling needs of people seeking regulated fertility treatment. This identified four main types of counselling:

- the provision of information (information counselling);
- the opportunity to reflect upon the procedures (implications counselling);
- the provision of emotional support (support counselling);
- the initiation of sustained help, if necessary, to enable individuals to adjust to particular life circumstances (therapeutic counselling).

6:4.1 Information counselling
This ensures individuals are given relevant information about:

- the risks and complications associated with the procedure;
- the likelihood of success or failure in their own case; and
- the rights and duties in relation to any child which might result and the possible impact on other children who may be affected.

6:4.2 Implications counselling
This is intended to enable individuals to explore some of the following:

- the impact and implications of infertility;
- their own motivations in seeking a surrogate mother or offering to be one;
- the implications of surrogacy as a way to form a family;
- their possible reactions to success or failure of treatment;

- other ways of dealing with childlessness, now, or later if treatment fails;
- the effect on the surrogate and on her family of parting with the child;
- how and what the child will be told of its origins;
- the implications of keeping secrets within a family; and
- the implications of maintaining a long-term relationship between intended parents and the surrogate mother and the complexities of such an arrangement.

If partial surrogacy is sought, implications counselling can help the intended mother to examine her feelings about raising a child genetically unrelated to her.

Unlike information counselling, which may come from many diverse sources, the BMA recommends that implications counselling should be provided only by a trained infertility counsellor.

6:4.3 Support counselling

This is intended to provide emotional support. Although specialised counsellors may be involved, the value of people such as friends, relatives, or individuals who have undergone similar experiences should not be under-estimated. Such support can be helpful throughout and beyond the treatment process to counter the stresses generated by it.

6:4.4 Therapeutic counselling

Prolonged therapeutic counselling may be necessary for some people, either as a result of difficulties associated with fertility or other problems which may be exacerbated by infertility and treatment, such as marital and psychosexual problems. Those in need of such counselling should be referred for appropriate specialist help. Therapeutic counselling should similarly be available to those who find that surrogacy is not able to fulfil their wish for a child.

The length, type and content of counselling should be determined by the individual needs of those concerned. In many cases it is useful to offer counselling individually or with relevant others, such as partners, parents or other close family members. No one should be obliged to accept counselling but the BMA recommends that serious consideration of the opportunity to receive specialised counselling is to be strongly encouraged.

7 Guidelines for Health Professionals

1. Surrogacy is an acceptable option of last resort in cases where it is impossible or highly undesirable for medical reasons for the intended mother to carry a child herself. In all cases the interests of the potential child must be paramount and the risks to the surrogate mother must be kept to a minimum.

2. Health professionals consulted about a surrogacy arrangement should inform themselves about the legal position before offering advice. In particular, health professionals should be aware of the non-enforceability of surrogacy arrangements and the legal position with regard to parentage of the child.

3. In surrogacy arrangements the level of the health professionals' ethical responsibilities will vary depending on the degree of involvement in the arrangement. The BMA has divided these into three broad categories: (i) health professionals consulted about an established pregnancy; (ii) those consulted by women considering self-insemination; and (iii) those professional teams providing assisted conception techniques for the establishment of a pregnancy involving a surrogacy arrangement. Health professionals have responsibilities to all their patients. However, where health professionals are providing treatment services to assist people to have children they have additional responsibilities to the potential child.

4. Once a surrogate pregnancy has been established, the practitioner's ethical obligations to the surrogate mother and child are no different from those owed to any other pregnant woman except that additional support may be required. The duty of the health care team is to provide the appropriate level of support and guidance both during and after the pregnancy.

5. Practitioners approached by people considering self-insemination should encourage those concerned to consider the issues and implications very carefully and should ensure that they are

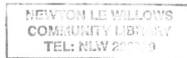
NEWTON LE WILLOWS
COMMUNITY LIBRARY
TEL: NLW 2____9

59

aware of how to obtain accurate information about the medical, psychological, emotional and legal issues involved with surrogacy.

6. Before agreeing to provide licensed treatment services aimed at establishing a surrogate pregnancy, for example through in vitro fertilisation or donor insemination, the health care team must take all reasonable steps to ensure that the medical, emotional and legal issues have been carefully considered and must, in all cases, take account of the welfare of the child who may be born as a result of the treatment. Such treatment services may only be provided in clinics licensed by the Human Fertilisation & Embryology Authority (HFEA) and in compliance with the HFEA's Code of Practice. Before proceeding with treatment, health professionals should also satisfy themselves that the intended parents have tried all other reasonable treatment options.

7. Some health professionals who are not providing treatment services or advising on surrogacy may nonetheless be aware that a woman is, or a couple are, considering surrogacy. In such cases, the practitioner should seek to persuade them to share relevant information which might be important to the overall assessment of the interests of the potential child. It is particularly important to divulge information, such as a history of child abuse or neglect, to the medical team providing the treatment services. If such information highlights an *exceptional* risk to the parties involved, the person should be informed that the practitioner might, in a rare and particularly serious case, consider disclosing such details without his or her consent. In such cases the person should first be advised of this intention and be given the opportunity to divulge the relevant information voluntarily, or to challenge the disclosure.

8. Health professionals providing treatment services or advice about surrogacy, should actively encourage those considering this option to seek counselling and testing for infectious diseases.

9. Health professionals providing advice or treatment services should also emphasise the importance of discussing with all parties, in advance, the decisions which may need to be made

before, during and after the pregnancy. These include decisions about the number of embryos to be replaced in surrogacy using IVF, the level of prenatal testing, the preferred method of delivery and decisions about care in the immediate postpartum period. Ideally these decisions should be reached by mutual agreement but in all cases of dispute, the surrogate mother, in conjunction with the health professionals, should make the final decision.

10. There should be mutual trust and openness between the health professionals and their patients as much as between the individual parties to the arrangement.

11. It is important that care and treatment are provided non-judgmentally.

12. The surrogate mother should usually have successfully borne at least one child prior to the surrogacy arrangement and preferably will have completed her own family and have a partner, family or friends to provide support throughout and after the pregnancy. In some cases, particular attention may be necessary where family support is to be given to the surrogate mother and the intended mother from the same family.

13. In view of the potential risks to the surrogate mother's health, the intended parents should be advised of the importance of ensuring that proper insurance cover has been arranged for the surrogate mother.

14. All of the health professionals involved should understand clearly who has overall management of the pregnancy.

15. After birth, the surrogate mother, her family and the intended parents are likely to need additional support and advice. These needs should be recognised by the health team. Midwives and health visitors have a particularly important role to play at this stage.

16. Health professionals providing treatment services aimed at establishing a surrogate pregnancy should ensure, before proceeding, that consideration has been given to the long-term medical and psychological needs of those participating in the arrangement.

17. Openness and truth-telling between parents and children is generally to be encouraged.

18. Health professionals with a conscientious objection to surrogacy are not obliged to participate in the arrangement but have an ethical duty to refer the patient to another practitioner who would be prepared to consider offering help and advice.

Surrogacy Arrangements Act 1985 (as amended)

1985 CHAPTER 49

An Act to regulate certain activities in connection with arrangements made with a view to women carrying children as surrogate mothers. [16th July 1985]

B E IT ENACTED by the Queen's most Excellent Majesty, by and with the advice and consent of the Lords Spiritual and Temporal, and Commons, in this present Parliament assembled, and by the authority of the same, as follows:-

Meaning of "surrogate mother", "surrogacy arrangement" and other terms.

1.—(1) The following provisions shall have effect for the interpretation of this Act.

(2) "Surrogate mother" means a woman who carries a child in pursuance of an arrangement
  (*a*) made before she began to carry the child, and
  (*b*) made with a view to any child carried in pursuance of it being handed over to, and the parental rights being exercised (so far as practicable) by, another person or other persons.

(3) An arrangement is a surrogacy arrangement if, were a woman to whom the arrangement relates to carry a child in pursuance of it, she would be a surrogate mother.

(4) In determining whether an arrangement is made with such a view as is mentioned in subsection (2) above regard may be had to the circumstances as a whole (and, in particular, where there is a promise or understanding that any payment will or may be made to the woman or for her benefit in respect of the carrying of any child in pursuance of the arrangement, to that promise or understanding).

(5) An arrangement may be regarded as made with such a view though subject to conditions relating to the handing over of any child.

(6) A woman who carries a child is to be treated for the purposes of subsection (2)(a) above as beginning to carry it at the time of the insemination or, of the placing in her of an embryo, of an egg in the process of fertilisation or of sperm and eggs, as the case may be.

(7) "Body of persons" means a body of persons corporate or unincorporate.

(8) "Payment" means payment in money or money's worth.

(9) This Act applies to arrangements whether or not they are lawful.

Surrogacy arrangements unenforceable.

1A.—No surrogacy arrangement is enforceable by or against any of the persons making it.

Negotiating surrogacy arrangements on a commercial basis, etc.

2.—(1) No person shall on a commercial basis do any of the following acts in the United Kingdom, that is—
  (a) initiate or take part in any negotiations with a view to the making of a surrogacy arrangement,
  (b) offer or agree to negotiate the making of a surrogacy arrangement, or
  (c) compile any information with a view to its use in making, or negotiating the making of, surrogacy arrangements;

and no person shall in the United Kingdom knowingly cause another to do any of those acts on a commercial basis.

(2) A person who contravenes subsection (1) above is guilty of an offence; but it is not a contravention of that subsection—

   (*a*) for a woman, with a view to becoming a surrogate mother herself, to do any act mentioned in that subsection or to cause such an act to be done, or

   (*b*) for any person, with a view to a surrogate mother carrying a child for him, to do such an act or to cause such an act to be done.

(3) For the purposes of this section, a person does an act on a commercial basis (subject to subsection (4) below) if—

   (*a*) any payment is at any time received by himself or another in respect of it, or

   (*b*) he does it with a view to any payment being received by himself or another in respect of making, or negotiating or facilitating the making of, any surrogacy arrangement.

In this subsection "payment" does not include payment to or for the benefit of a surrogate mother or prospective surrogate mother.

(4) In proceedings against a person for an offence under subsection (1) above, he is not to be treated as doing an act on a commercial basis by reason of any payment received by another in respect of the act if it is proved that—

   (*a*) in a case where the payment was received before he did the act, he did not do the act knowing or having reasonable cause to suspect that any payment had been received in respect of the act; and

   (*b*) in any other case, he did not do the act with a view to any payment being received in respect of it.

(5) Where—

   (*a*) a person acting on behalf of a body of persons takes any part in negotiating or facilitating the making of a surrogacy arrangement in the United Kingdom, and

   (*b*) negotiating or facilitating the making of surrogacy arrangements is an activity of the body,

then, if the body at any time receives any payment made by or on behalf of—

      (i) a woman who carries a child in pursuance of the arrangement,

   (ii) the person or persons for whom she carries it,
or
   (iii) any person connected with the woman or with
   that person or those persons,

the body is guilty of an offence.

For the purposes of this subsection, a payment received by a person connected with a body is to be treated as received by the body.

(6) In proceedings against a body for an offence under subsection (5) above, it is a defence to prove that the payment concerned was not made in respect of the arrangement mentioned in paragraph (*a*) of that subsection.

(7) A person who in the United Kingdom takes part in the management or control—
   (*a*) of any body of persons, or
   (*b*) of any of the activities of any body of persons,
is guilty of an offence if the activity described in subsection (8) below is an activity of the body concerned.

(8) The activity referred to in subsection (7) above is negotiating or facilitating the making of surrogacy arrangements in the United Kingdom, being—
   (*a*) arrangements the making of which is negotiated or facilitated on a commercial basis, or
   (*b*) arrangements in the case of which payments are received (or treated for the purposes of subsection (5) above as received) by the body concerned in contravention of subsection (5) above.

(9) In proceedings against a person for an offence under subsection (7) above, it is a defence to prove that he neither knew nor had reasonable cause to suspect that the activity described in subsection (8) above was an activity of the body concerned; and for the purposes of such proceedings any arrangement falling within subsection (8)(*b*) above shall be disregarded if it is proved that the payment concerned was not made in respect of the arrangement.

Advertisements about surrogacy.

3.—(1) This section applies to any advertisement containing an indication (however expressed)—

(*a*) that any person is or may be willing to enter into a surrogacy arrangement or to negotiate or facilitate the making of a surrogacy arrangement, or

(*b*) that any person is looking for a woman willing to become a surrogate mother or for persons wanting a woman to carry a child as a surrogate mother.

(2) Where a newspaper or periodical containing an advertisement to which this section applies is published in the United Kingdom, any proprietor, editor or publisher of the newspaper or periodical is guilty of an offence.

(3) Where an advertisement to which this section applies is conveyed by means of a telecommunication system so as to be seen or heard (or both) in the United Kingdom, any person who in the United Kingdom causes it to be so conveyed knowing it to contain such an indication as is mentioned in subsection (1) above is guilty of an offence.

(4) A person who publishes or causes to be published in the United Kingdom an advertisement to which this section applies (not being an advertisement contained in a newspaper or periodical or conveyed by means of a telecommunication system) is guilty of an offence.

(5) A person who distributes or causes to be distributed in the United Kingdom an advertisement to which this section applies (not being an advertisement contained in a newspaper or periodical published outside the United Kingdom or an advertisement conveyed by means of a telecommunication system) knowing it to contain such an indication as is mentioned in subsection (1) above is guilty of an offence.

84 c.12.   (6) In this section "telecommunication system" has the same meaning as in the Telecommunications Act 1984.

Offences

4.—(1) A person guilty of an offence under this Act shall be liable on summary conviction—

(a) in the case of an offence under section 2 to a fine not exceeding level 5 on the standard scale or to imprisonment for a term not exceeding 3 months or both,

(b) in the case of an offence under section 3 to a fine not exceeding level 5 on the standard scale.

In this subsection "the standard scale" has the meaning given by section 75 of the Criminal Justice Act 1982.   1982 c

(2) No proceedings for an offence under this Act shall be instituted—

(a) in England and Wales, except by or with the consent of the Director of Public Prosecutions; and

(b) in Northern Ireland, except by or with the consent of the Director of Public Prosecutions for Northern Ireland.

(3) Where an offence under this Act committed by a body corporate is proved to have been committed with the consent or connivance of, or to be attributable to any neglect on the part of, any director, manager, secretary or other similar officer of the body corporate or any person who was purporting to act in any such capacity, he as well as the body corporate is guilty of the offence and is liable to be proceeded against and punished accordingly.

(4) Where the affairs of a body corporate are managed by its members, subsection (3) above shall apply in relation to the acts and defaults of a member in connection with his functions of management as if he were a director of the body corporate.

(5) In any proceedings for an offence under section 2 of this Act, proof of things done or of words written, spoken or published (whether or not in the presence of any party to the proceedings) by any person taking part in the management or control of a body of persons or of any of the activities of the body, or by any person doing any of the acts mentioned in subsection (1)(a) to (c) of that section on behalf of the body, shall be admissible as evidence of the activities of the body.

(6) In relation to an offence under this Act, section 127(1) of the Magistrates' Courts Act 1980 (information must be laid within six   1980 c.4 months of commission of offence), section 331(1) of the Criminal Procedure (Scotland) Act 1975 (proceedings must be commenced   1975 c.2 within that time) and Article 19(1) of the Magistrates'

S1/1675
5). Courts (Northern Ireland) Order 1981 (complaint must be made within that time) shall have effect as if for the reference to six months there were substituted a reference to two years.

Short title and extent.

5.—(1) This Act may be cited as the Surrogacy Arrangements Act 1985.

(2) This Act extends to Northern Ireland.

References

1. Bromham D, *Public Acceptance of Surrogacy: What are the Limits?* (Abstract 0698) in Ratnam S, Teoh E, Seng K & Macnaughton M (eds) <u>Proceedings of the Thirteenth World Congress of Gynaecology and Obstetrics (FIGO)</u> (1991) Abstracts 3 pp.305-314. Elsevier, New York.

2. Morgan D, *Surrogacy: An Introductory Essay* in Lee RG & Morgan D (eds) <u>Birthrights. Law and Ethics at the Beginning of Life</u> (1989) and Morgan D, *A Surrogacy Issue: Who is the Other Mother?* (1994) 8 International Journal of Law & The Family 386.

3. *Report of the Committee of Inquiry into Human Fertilisation and Embryology*, HMSO, Cmnd 9314, July 1984, paras 2.5-2.13.

4. Freeman MDA, *Is Surrogacy Exploitative?* in McLean S (ed) <u>Legal Issues in Human Reproduction</u> (1989) Aldershot, Dartmouth.

5. The complexities of the Adoption Act 1976 in relation to surrogacy are discussed by Douglas G, *Law, Fertility and Reproduction* (1991) pp.161-162.

6. Capron A, *Alternative Birth Technologies: Legal Challenges* (1987) 20 Univ. California Davis Law Rev. 697.

7. *Human Fertilisation and Embryology Act 1990*, HMSO, sections 12-15.

8. Section 36 of the Human Fertilisation and Embryology Act inserts section 1A in the Surrogacy Arrangements Act 1985 and provides that "No surrogacy arrangement is enforceable by or against any of the persons making it".

9. *Human Fertilisation and Embryology Act 1990*, HMSO, section 27.

10. Ibid, section 28.

11. For a detailed discussion of these provisions see Morgan D and

Lee RG, *Blackstone's Guide to the Human Fertilisation and Embryology Act 1990*, (1991) Blackstone Press, London pp.154-156.

12. *Human Fertilisation and Embryology Act 1990*, HMSO, section 13(5).

13. Human Fertilisation & Embryology Authority, *Code of Practice* (1993), para 3.16.

14. Ibid, para 3.15.

15. Ibid, para 3.33.

16. Evidence provided to the Steering Group by COTS (Childlessness Overcome Through Surrogacy).

17. A useful discussion of the advantages and disadvantages of clinical ethics committees can be found in Thornton JG, Lilford RJ, *Clinical Ethics Committees*, BMJ, 1995, vol 311 pp.667-669.

18. Human Fertilisation & Embryology Authority, *Fourth Annual Report* (1995) p.31.

19. The *Report on Confidential Enquiries into Maternal Deaths in the United Kingdom 1988-1990* is discussed in Department of Health *On the State of the Public Health 1994* (1995) HMSO, London.

20. Sleep J, Grant A, Garcia J, Elbourne D, Spencer J, Chalmers I, *West Berkshire Perineal Management Trial* (1984) BMJ Clinical Research 289 (6445) pp.587-590.

21. Glazener CM, Abdalla M, Stroud P, Naji S, Templeton A, Russell IT, *Postnatal Maternal Morbidity: Extent, Causes, Prevention and Treatment* (1995) British Journal of Obstetrics & Gynaecology 102 (4) pp.282-287.

22. Stratton P, *Does Surrogacy Raise Major Psychological Problems?* (1990) Bulletin of the Society for Reproductive and Infant Psychology 11.

23. Blyth E, *Section 30 - the Acceptable Face of Surrogacy?* (1993) Journal of Social Welfare and Family Law 4 pp.248-260.

24. Parker PJ, *Motivation of Surrogate Mothers: Initial Findings* (1983) American Journal of Psychiatry 140(1) pp.117-118.

25. Fischer S & Gillman I, *Surrogate Motherhood: Attachment, Attitudes and Social Support* (1991) Psychiatry 54 pp.13-20.

26. Franks D, *Psychiatric Evaluation of Women in a Surrogate Mother Program* (1981) American Journal of Psychiatry 138(10) pp.1378-1379.

27. MacPhee D & Forest K, *Surrogacy: Programme Comparisons and Policy Implications* (1990) International Journal of Law & The Family 4 pp.308-317.

28. Reame N & Parker P, *Surrogate Pregnancy: Clinical Features of 44 Cases* (1983) American Journal of Obstetrics & Gynaecology 162 pp.1220-1225.

29. Einwohner J, *Who Becomes a Surrogate. Personality Characteristics* (1989) in Offerman-Zuckerberg J (ed) Gender in Transition. A New Frontier. Plenum Publishing Corporation, New York.

30. Reame NE, *Maternal Adaptation and Postpartum Responses to a Surrogate Pregnancy* (1989) Abstracts of the 9th International Congress of Psychosomatic Obstetrics & Gynaecology. Journal of Psychosomatic Obstetrics & Gynaecology 10 (Supplement 1).

31. Schmukler I & Aigen BP, *The Terror of Surrogate Motherhood. Fantasies, Realities and Viable Legislation* (1989) in Offerman-Zuckerberg J (ed) Gender in Transition. A New Frontier. Plenum Publishing Corporation, New York.

32. Evidence provided to the Steering Group by COTS (Childlessness Overcome Through Surrogacy).

33. *Human Fertilisation and Embryology Act 1990*, HMSO, section 13(6).

34. King's Fund Counselling Committee, *Counselling for Regulated Infertility Treatments* (1991). King's Fund Centre, London.

Index